ON CALL
PSYCHIATRY

Haldol 5   10
Ativan 2   4
Cogentin ½ 1

Be ON CALL with confidence!

Successfully managing on-call situations requires a masterful combination of speed, skill, and knowledge. Rise to the occasion with **W.B. SAUNDERS' On Call Series!** These pocket-size resources provide you with immediate access to the vital, step-by-step information you need to succeed!

Other Titles in the On Call Series

ON CALL
PSYCHIATRY
Second Edition

Carol A. Bernstein, MD
Associate Professor of Clinical Psychiatry
Director of Residency Training
Department of Psychiatry
New York University School of Medicine
New York, New York

Waguih William IsHak, MD
Research Assistant Professor of Psychiatry
Department of Psychiatry
New York University of School of Medicine
New York, New York

Elyse D. Weiner, MD
Clinical Assistant Professor of Psychiatry
Department of Psychiatry
New York University School of Medicine
New York, New York

Brian J. Ladds, MD
Adjunct Faculty
New York University School of Medicine
Saint Vincent's Hospital
New York, New York

W.B. SAUNDERS COMPANY
An Imprint of Elsevier Science
Philadelphia   London   New York   St. Louis   Sydney   Toronto

W.B. SAUNDERS COMPANY
An Imprint of Elsevier Science

The Curtis Center
Independence Square West
Philadelphia, Pennsylvania 19106

Library of Congress Cataloging-in-Publication Data

On call psychiatry / [edited by] Carol A. Bernstein . . . [et al.].—2nd ed.

p.   cm.

Includes bibliographical references and index.

ISBN 0–7216–9239–7

1. Psychiatric emergencies.   2. Crisis intervention (Mental health services)   I. Bernstein, Carol A.   [DNLM: 1. Crisis Intervention. 2. Emergency Services, Psychiatric.   WM 401 O58 2001]

RC480.6 .O5 2001   616.89′025—dc21

2001020322

Acquisitions Editor: William Schmitt
Manuscript Editor: Amy Norwitz
Production Manager: Norman Stellander
Illustration Specialist: John Needles
Book Designer: Matt Andrews

ON CALL PSYCHIATRY   ISBN 0–7216–9239–7

Printed in the United States of America.

Last digit is the print number: 9   8   7   6   5   4   3   2

In memory of Douglas E. Fogelman, MD, who practiced medicine in the true spirit of Hippocrates.

CONTRIBUTORS

Note: At the time of writing, all of the contributors were residents in the Adult Psychiatry Training Program at New York University Medical Center.

Ava Albrecht, MD
Clinical Instructor
Department of Psychiatry
New York University School
  of Medicine
New York, New York
*The Emergency Evaluation of
  Children and Adolescents;
  Physical and Behavioral
  Indicators of Abuse*

Sean Allan, MD
Consultation Liaison Fellow
Department of Psychiatry
New York University School
  of Medicine
New York, New York
Insomnia

**Khleber Chapman Attwell,
MD, MPH**
PGY4 Resident and Chief
  Resident
Department of Psychiatry
New York University School
  of Medicine
New York, New York
*The Approach to Emergency
  Psychiatric Diagnosis; The
  Suicidal Patient*

Jonathan Bellman, MD
PGY4 Resident
Department of Psychiatry
New York University School
  of Medicine
New York, New York
Urine Toxicology; Medication

*Levels; Clonidine
  Detoxification Protocol for
  Opioid Dependence*

Scott Bienenfeld, MD
PGY4 Resident
Department of Psychiatry
New York University School
  of Medicine
New York, New York
*Intoxication; Substance
  Withdrawal; Detoxification
  Protocol for Alcohol
  Dependence*

Hillery Bosworth, MD
PGY4 Resident and Chief
  Resident
Department of Psychiatry
New York University School
  of Medicine
New York, New York
On Call Formulary

Brian Bronson, MD
PGY4 Resident and Chief
  Resident
Department of Psychiatry
New York University School
  of Medicine
New York, New York
*Mutism and Other Problems
  With Speech and
  Communication*

**Madeleine Castellanos,
MD**
PGY4 Resident
Department of Psychiatry

New York University School
of Medicine
New York, New York
Headache; Nausea and Vomiting

Christine Desmond, MD
Clinical Instructor
Department of Psychiatry
New York University School
of Medicine
New York, New York
*The Psychotic Patient; Common
Adverse Effects of Psychotropic
Medications*

Sharon Falco, MD
Clinical Instructor
Department of Psychiatry
New York University School
of Medicine
New York, New York
*The Psychotic Patient; Common
Adverse Effects of Psychotropic
Medications*

Mara Goldstein, MD
PGY4 Resident and Chief
Resident
Department of Psychiatry
New York University School
of Medicine
New York, New York
*Seclusion and Restraint;
Assessment of Competency and
Other Legal Issues*

Ceri E. Hadda, MD
PGY5 Resident
Geriatric Psychiatry
Mt. Sinai School of Medicine
New York, New York
*The Confused Patient: Delirium
and Dementia; Elder Abuse
and Neglect*

Markus J. Kraebber, MD
PGY3 Resident
Department of Psychiatry

New York University School
of Medicine
New York, New York
Fever; Blood Pressure Changes

Mark Krushelnycky, MD
PGY5 Resident
Department of Child
Psychiatry
New York University School
of Medicine
New York, New York
*The Emergency Evaluation of
Children and Adolescents;
Physical and Behavioral
Indicators of Abuse*

**Michelle E. Montemayor,
MD, PhD**
Clinical Instructor
Department of Psychiatry
New York University School
of Medicine
New York, New York
*The Difficult Patient; The Violent
Patient*

Siddhartha Nadkarni, MD
PGY4 Resident
Department of Psychiatry
New York University School
of Medicine
New York, New York
*Falls; Mental Status
Examination; The Neurologic
Examination*

Adam Raff, MD
PGY4 Resident
Department of Psychiatry
New York University School
of Medicine
New York, New York
*Rigidity and Neuroleptic
Malignant Syndrome*

Noah L. Rosen, MD
PGY4 Resident
Department of Psychiatry
New York University School
   of Medicine
New York, New York
*Falls; Mental Status
   Examination; The
   Neurologic Examination*

Julie K. Schulman, MD
Consultation Liaison Fellow
Department of Psychiatry
New York Presbyterian
   Hospital
New York, New York
*The Role of the Psychiatric
   Consultant; Telephone
   Consultations*

Ira L. Scott, Jr., MD
PGY3 Resident
Department of Psychiatry
New York University School
   of Medicine
New York, New York
Chest Pain

M. Brealyn Sellers, MD
PGY4 Resident
Department of Psychiatry
New York University School
   of Medicine
New York, New York
*Intoxication; Substance
   Withdrawal; Clonidine
   Detoxification Protocol for
   Opioid Dependence;
   Detoxification Protocol for
   Alcohol Dependence*

Erwin C. Ting, MD
Consultation Liaison Fellow
Department of Psychiatry
Beth Israel Medical Center
New York, New York
*Seizures; Normal Laboratory
   Values; Important Telephone
   Numbers*

Elisabeth Weinstein, MD
PGY4 Resident
Department of Psychiatry
New York University School
   of Medicine
New York, New York
The Agitated Patient

Steven Wozniak, MD
Attending Psychiatrist
Department of Psychiatry
Woodhull Hospital Center
Brooklyn, New York
*Medical Conditions Manifesting
   as Psychiatric Disorders*

Patrick Ying, MD
PGY4 Resident and Chief
   Resident
Department of Psychiatry
New York University School
   of Medicine
New York, New York
*The Anxious Patient; On Call
   Formulary*

Van Yu, MD
Clinical Instructor
Department of Psychiatry
New York University School
   of Medicine
New York, New York
*Physical and Sexual Trauma;
   Admission Orders*

FOREWORD

The experience of being on call is the traditional rite of passage for physicians undergoing specialty training. In the arena of the unexpected, trainees have for centuries honed key skills, acquired essential knowledge, and developed the calm and reassuring attitudes associated with superb physicianhood.

The challenges of emergency calls in psychiatry are growing exponentially as a result of the vast changes occurring in our health care systems. Patients are admitted to inpatient care today far sicker than ever before. The presence of significant medical and substance abuse co-morbidities complicates emergency decision making and requires expanding knowledge of differential diagnoses and therapeutic techniques.

The dramatic expansion of pharmacology in general and psychopharmacology in particular requires of the on-call psychiatrist an awareness of drug–drug interactions and knowledge of the potential psychogenic impact of the myriad medications used in medical practice.

The medicolegal context for the practice of medicine and psychiatry is also changing. Decisions such as the use of restraint and seclusion, formally governed largely by clinical judgment, are now mired in complex and restrictive regulations.

For all these reasons, the on-call experience of trainees must be supported by explicit knowledge and careful supervision. In this spirit, the authors of this text articulate and distill their vast emergency experience into concise action plans.

The text covers the on-call situation from different angles. First, patient-related diagnostic problems such as agitation, anxiety, and psychosis are covered in an immediately usable, practical fashion. Second, the ever-expanding boundary between psychiatry and medicine is addressed as the authors discuss problems such as seizures and neuroleptic malignant syndrome with reassuring clarity. Finally, careful attention is paid to framing optimal clinical and medicolegal approaches to problems such as competency assessment, use of restraint and seclusion, abuse and neglect, and physical and sexual trauma.

I am confident that, aided by this book, the postgraduate trainee will be able to provide his or her patient with superb and compassionate emergency care. The authors should be commended for passing on, with such ease, the knowledge and experience gained from trying to heal the awesome variety of human suffering presenting to psychiatric trainees. That the authors, all early in the development of their careers, exude the confidence and competence of veterans is a tribute to the educational value of well-supervised direct exposure to many diverse clinical situations of uncommon difficulty.

Manuel Trujillo, MD
Professor of Clinical Psychiatry
Vice-Chair, Department of Psychiatry
New York University School of Medicine
Director of Psychiatry
Bellevue Hospital Center
New York, New York

PREFACE

On Call Psychiatry has been developed by the psychiatric house-staff at the New York University School of Medicine as a resource guide for clinicians who are required to deal with psychiatric emergencies while on call. It distills the knowledge of psychiatric residents who have collectively spent thousands of hours on call at Bellevue Hospital Center, New York University Medical Center, and its affiliate hospitals. We are extremely pleased to have edited the second edition of *On Call Psychiatry*. We have retained our situational approach to the organization of this book because we are aware that psychiatric signs and symptoms are frequently significant long before the patient's diagnosis has become clear. We hope that this book will continue to serve as a practical manual for psychiatrists and other mental health professionals, as well as for physicians from other disciplines. We look forward to your comments, which add to the growth of *On Call Psychiatry* as a collective work.

We would like to thank Ann S. Maloney, MD, who resigned her editorship for this edition. We are in debt to her for bringing the idea to the residency program with the aid of W.B. Saunders as well as for her hard work and dedication on the first edition. We are delighted to welcome Waguih William IsHak, MD, who was a contributor to the first edition, as a co-editor on this edition. We would also like to sincerely thank our first group of contributors whose tireless writing and rewriting laid the foundation for this manuscript. We are indebted to Robert Cancro, MD, Lucius N. Littauer Professor and Chairman of the Department of Psychiatry at the New York University School of Medicine; and to Manuel Trujillo, MD, Director of Psychiatry at Bellevue Hospital Center, for their ongoing support. We would also like to acknowledge the invaluable support of our friends and families as well as our faculty and supervisors, who have been a consistent resource. Finally, we are deeply grateful to our patients, who are our finest teachers and without whom none of this would be possible.

Carol A. Bernstein
Waguih William IsHak
Elyse D. Weiner
Brian J. Ladds

NOTICE

Psychiatry is an ever-changing field. Standard safety precautions must be followed, but as new research and clinical experience broaden our knowledge, changes in treatment and drug therapy become necessary or appropriate. Readers are advised to check the most current product information provided by the manufacturer of each drug to be administered to verify the recommended dose, the method and duration of administration, and the contraindications. It is the responsibility of the treating physician, relying on experience and knowledge of the patient, to determine dosages and the best treatment for each individual patient. Neither the publisher nor the editor assumes any liability for any injury and/or damage to persons or property arising from this publication.

THE PUBLISHER

STRUCTURE OF THE BOOK

The book is divided into two main sections.

Section I covers introductory material in five chapters: (1) Approach to Emergency Psychiatric Diagnosis, (2) Role of the Psychiatric Consultant, (3) Telephone Consultations, (4) Seclusion and Restraint, and (5) Assessment of Competency and Other Legal Issues.

Section II contains the common calls associated with patient-related problems. Each problem is approached from its inception, beginning with the relevant questions that should be asked over the phone, the temporary orders that should be given, and the major life-threatening problems to be considered as one approaches the bedside:

■ PHONE CALLS

Questions

Pertinent questions to assess the urgency of the situation.

Orders

Urgent orders to be carried out before the housestaff arrives at the bedside.

Inform RN

RN to be informed of the time the housestaff anticipates arrival at the bedside.

■ ELEVATOR THOUGHTS

The possibilities in the differential diagnosis to be considered by the housestaff while on the way to assess the patient (i.e., while in the elevator).

■ MAJOR THREAT TO LIFE

Identification of the major threat to life is essential in providing focus for the subsequent effective management of the patient.

■ BEDSIDE

Quick Look Test

The quick look test is a rapid visual assessment to place the patient into one of three categories: well, sick, or critical. This helps determine the necessity for immediate intervention.

Vital Signs

Selective History and Chart Review

Selective Physical Examination

■ MANAGEMENT

The Appendices consist of reference items that we have found useful in managing calls.

The On Call Formulary is a compendium of commonly used medications that are likely to be prescribed by the student or resident on call. The formulary serves as a quick, alphabetically arranged reference for indications, drug dosages, routes of administration, side effects, contraindications, and modes of action.

COMMONLY USED ABBREVIATIONS

ADHD	attention-deficit/hyperactivity disorder
AFB	acid-fast bacilli
AIDS	acquired immunodeficiency syndrome
ALT	alanine aminotransferase
ANA	antinuclear antibody
APA	American Psychiatric Association
AST	aspartate transaminase
BID	twice a day
BP	blood pressure
BUN	blood urea nitrogen
CBC	complete blood count
CHF	congestive heart failure
CISD	Critical Incident Stress Debriefing
CK	creatine kinase
CNS	central nervous system
COPD	chronic obstructive pulmonary disease
CPAP	continuous positive airway pressure
CSAS	central sleep apnea syndrome
CSF	cerebrospinal fluid
CT	computed tomography
CVA	cerebrovascular accident
DNR	Do not resuscitate
DSM-III-R	*Diagnostic and Statistical Manual of Mental Disorders*, 3rd Edition, Revised
DSM-IV	*Diagnostic and Statistical Manual of Mental Disorders*, 4th Edition
DTs	delirium tremens

DVT	deep vein thrombosis
ECG	electrocardiogram
ECT	electroconvulsive therapy
EEG	electroencephalogram
EMG	electromyogram
EPS	extrapyramidal symptoms
ER	emergency room
ERCP	endoscopic retrograde cholangiopancreatography
ESR	erythrocyte sedimentation rate
ETOH	ethanol (alcohol)
GABA	gamma-aminobutyric acid
GAD	generalized anxiety disorder
GGT	gamma-glutamyltransferase
GI	gastrointestinal
HEENT	head, eyes, ears, nose, and throat
HIV	human immunodeficiency virus
HPI	history of present illness
HR	heart rate
HS	half-strength
IM	intramuscular
IV	intravenous
LAAM	L-acetyl-alpha-methadol
LD	laryngeal dystonia
LDH	lactate dehydrogenase
LFT	liver function test
LP	lumbar puncture
LSD	lysergic acid diethylamide
MAO	monoamine oxidase
MAOI	monoamine oxidase inhibitor
MI	myocardial infarction
MRI	magnetic resonance imaging

MSE	mental status examination
NA	Narcotics Anonymous
NMS	neuroleptic malignant syndrome
NS	normal saline
NSAID	nonsteroidal anti-inflammatory drug
1PC	certification by one physician
OBG	obstetrician-gynecologist
OCD	obsessive-compulsive disorder
OSAS	obstructive sleep apnea syndrome
PCP	phencyclidine hydrochloride
PE	pulmonary embolism
PLMD	periodic limb movement disorder
PO	per os (by mouth)
PRN	as necessary
PTSD	post-traumatic stress disorder
PVC	premature ventricular contraction
QD	every day
QHS	at bedtime
QID	four times a day
RBC	red blood cell count
REM	rapid eye movement
RLS	restless legs syndrome
RPR	rapid plasma reagin
SC	subcutaneous
SIADH	syndrome of inappropriate antidiuretic hormone
SLE	systemic lupus erythematosus
SSRI	selective serotonin reuptake inhibitor
2PC	certification by two physicians
T_3	triiodothyronine
T_4	thyroxine
T_3RU	triiodothyronine resin uptake

TB	tuberculosis
TBG	thyroxine-binding globulin
TCA	tricyclic antidepressant
TID	three times a day
TMJ	temporomandibular joint
TN	transdermal nicotine
TRH	thyrotropin-releasing hormone
TSH	thyroid-stimulating hormone
U/A	urinalysis
UTI	urinary tract infection

CONTENTS

APPENDICES

INTRODUCTION

1 | The Approach to Emergency Psychiatric Diagnosis

KHLEBER CHAPMAN ATTWELL

Welcome to Psychiatric Emergency; whether you consult this book in a small town's general hospital ward on call or in the thick of a major metropolitan psychiatric emergency room equipped with fully trained staff, the principles remain the same. The emergent task at hand becomes that of triage, evaluation, formulation, and disposition, keeping safety for the patient, others, and oneself always at the forefront. Once the patient is safe and correctly situated, thorough inpatient/outpatient assessment can follow. Whether you are faced with a labile man in restraints or a late-night sandwich seeker, your job becomes detective in nature: What caused this person to come here, and how can you be of help? Even if the patient is "only asking for a sandwich," you must ask why he or she has chosen the psychiatric emergency room to do so. A careful, systematic approach can make good work practice routine, missing no detail. Appropriate management of psychiatric emergencies saves lives.

Safety first. Always judge this for yourself. If the patient makes you uncomfortable in the slightest, pay attention. Order chemical or physical restraints and defer the interview until you feel comfortable; or leave the interview to get security backup. Interview the patient with police if necessary; order as-needed medication and restraints over the phone before seeing the patient if such is indicated and you think the patient might become agitated before your assessment. Do not think twice about ordering a one-to-one watch until more stable arrangements can be made. You can always take a patient out of restraints later or cancel a one-to-one watch; it is more difficult to bring the patient's body back in the window or restore your fellow staff member's jaw to normal after the fact. Resist all attempts by administrators or nurses to avoid one-to-one observation if doing so is in the patient's best interest. Most staff members understand the need for close observation if provided reasons simply and calmly. Likewise, resist any urge to handle a dangerous patient on your own; once the door is shut behind you, it may be too late. It is your job to ensure safety for all involved.

Second, triage. With what level of severity are you dealing? Is the patient arousable and alert, with stable vital signs? You do not want to miss the accidental heroin overdose or an evolving delirium tremens. If you suspect any potentially dangerous physical abnormality, involve your medical colleagues promptly. After ruling out life-threatening emergencies, which would require emergent transfer, perform a medical evaluation. Many seemingly less acute consults or presentations involve infectious processes, pulmonary conditions, pain, laboratory abnormalities, hemorrhage, or adverse drug reactions. Check medications, vital signs, laboratory data, and radiologic evidence for medical causes of psychiatric morbidity. Abnormal vital signs should lead you to consider infection, cardiovascular abnormalities, withdrawal syndromes, poisoning, neuroleptic malignant syndrome, or toxicities of medication. Electrolyte abnormalities may induce mental status changes, as can central nervous system (CNS) events, withdrawals, and infections. Liver pathology invites a consideration of alcohol-related disease and hepatic encephalopathy. When available, check thyroid function, B_{12}/folate levels, rapid plasma reagin (RPR), and urine toxicology. Numerous medications can affect the CNS, so review the patient's current medication regimen.

Once you have guaranteed safety and thoroughly ruled out medical causes for the presentation, consider psychiatric disorders. What does the patient look like? What is the history, and are you able to gather one in conjunction with your mental status examination? What makes the patient present now? Why has the house staff chosen this moment to call for help? Has some covert acute stressor occurred—the breakup of a relationship, the death of a loved one, a pending vacation or family reunion? Have drugs and alcohol played a part in the decompensation? Has some environmental change (loss of luggage or of housing) led to a loss of medication?

A word about collateral sources of information. Histories provided by psychiatric patients may skew events into delusional proportions or provide accounts inconsistent with those of other observers. Family members, former psychiatrists, old medical records/discharge summaries, case managers, and nursing staff on the patient's floor can prove invaluable, particularly when the patient wishes to deny all past psychiatric history in order to avoid admission to the hospital. Call collateral sources; interview friends and relatives at the bedside; talk with those accompanying the patient; get a translator via the AT&T Language Bank should none be available in your hospital. Your interventions are only as effective as your history taking; a medical emergency is a valid reason for waking someone up in the middle of the night.

The patient's rate of decompensation can prove useful. Acute changes suggest medical illness or withdrawal syndromes; psychotic breaks with reality testing may develop over weeks to months, especially when medication may obscure symptoms.

A competent mental status examination provides not only rationale for treatments implemented but also a snapshot of the patient at a particular point in time, thereby allowing for the establishment of longitudinal benchmarks for all staff involved in the care of the patient. The mental status examination may prove vital in assessing the need for renewal of one-to-one watches or the diagnosis of delirium or intoxication. Tailor your examinations to the demands of the differential diagnosis at hand. Alcoholic patients require assessment of orientation; depressed patients deserve several questions exploring suicidal ideation; elderly or demented patients merit subtle inquiries into explorations of both cognitive function and decisional capacity. **Always** touch upon the following and avoid using abbreviations where possible:

- Patient's appearance
- Relatedness to interviewer and degree of cooperation
- Level of activity and agitation
- Mood and affect, with particular attention to lability
- Thought process
- Suicidal or homicidal ideation
- Psychotic dimensions of thought
- Brief cognitive examination, including level of alertness and orientation
- Insight and judgment

A thorough mental status examination will guide diagnosis and sound care. Delirious patients require medical attention; suicidal patients demand protection; labile patients may need chemical or physical restraint; psychosis often impairs decision-making capacity and ability to care for self; florid paranoia can endanger those in the community.

The full range of psychiatric symptomatology and diagnosis makes our job fascinating; keeping this in mind enables us to provide care in an appropriate, safe manner. Developing a sound differential diagnosis helps ensure the provision of competent care for the patient with abnormal behavior. Thorough understanding of mental illness comes only with time and detailed evaluation and study; in the emergency setting, however, the focus is the immediate assessment and provision of a safe channel for management and diagnosis of the situation at hand. Always err on the side of caution; interventions made during psychiatric emergencies can save lives as powerfully as in any specialty of medicine.

2 | The Role of the Psychiatric Consultant

JULIE K. SCHULMAN

The on-call physician may be asked by medical or surgical colleagues to consult about a patient on their service. This chapter addresses the issues involved in consultation.

■ BEING AN EFFECTIVE CONSULTANT

Your job as a psychiatric consultant is exciting, intellectually challenging, and also unpredictable. You may be called to see a patient for long-standing psychiatric illness, new psychiatric complaints, or a sudden change in mental status. At times, you will be called to see a patient not because of the patient's distress, but because of the distress the patient's behavior has generated in the treatment team, such as frustration or anger owing to the patient's repeated medical complaints.

The role you play has two aspects: your relationship with the patient and your relationship with the primary physician and treatment team. In your relationship with the patient, remember that in most cases you are there to provide a one-time evaluation only and that follow-up care will be provided by the regular consult-liaison team. The relationship between the consulting physician and the patient is limited to achieving the goal of the consult. Some patients may be resistant to the idea of seeing a psychiatrist, particularly if they had not been notified in advance by the requesting physician that a psychiatric consultation was ordered and told the reasons for the consultation.

Because the time spent with the patient usually will be brief, it is especially important to be aware of countertransference reactions in both the treating team and yourself. Dying patients may induce avoidance reactions because of feelings of helplessness, hopelessness, and identification with the patient. Patients with multiple somatic complaints, especially pain, or unexplained physical symptoms, hypochondriasis, and malingering may induce angry reactions secondary to frustration. Patients who are pleasant, attractive, intelligent, or successful may induce identification and overprotective feelings that may lead to minimization of psychiatric symptoms. Awareness of countertransference is crucial in handling difficult situations. You should maintain a professional demeanor and focus on the distressing issues that are manageable, such as the identification and treatment of depressive symptoms.

In your interactions with the primary physician and team, remember to listen carefully to what they have to tell you about their observations, as this information will be invaluable in your assessment. Although you are there primarily to provide recommendations for the patient's treatment, you can also play a valuable role in educating the medical team about countertransference reactions and other psychiatric issues related to medical care.

■ REASONS FOR CONSULTATION

The most common requests for consultation involve the following categories of psychiatric diagnoses.

Psychiatric Disorders due to Medical Conditions

- Delirium, dementia, amnesia, and other cognitive disorders
- Psychotic disorder due to a general medical condition
- Mood or anxiety disorder due to a general medical condition
- Mental disorder not otherwise specified due to a general medical condition

Psychiatric Disorders Manifesting as Medical Conditions

- Somatization or undifferentiated somatoform disorder
- Conversion disorder
- Factitious disorder
- Malingering

Psychiatric Disorders Related to Adjustment to Medical Conditions

- Adjustment disorder with depressed or anxious mood
- Psychologic factors affecting medical condition

Psychiatric Disorders Manifesting as Management Problems

- Any psychiatric disorder with suicidal or violent threats or behavior
- Personality disorders
- Assessment of decision-making capacity ("competency")

Substance-Related Disorders

- Intoxication
- Withdrawal
- Substance-induced psychiatric disorder

Other Psychiatric Disorders

- Any pre-existing psychiatric disorder (e.g., schizophrenia)
- Mental retardation or developmental disorder
- Sleep disorders

■ PHONE CALL

Questions

1. **How urgent is the situation?**

   Is there any immediate danger to the patient, the staff, or others? Is the patient suicidal or homicidal?

2. **What questions does the requesting physician want answered?**

   For all consults, except in emergencies, you need to speak directly to the physician ordering the consult. The requesting physician should give you a very brief history of the patient, including reason for admission, current medical status, presence or absence of substance abuse or known psychiatric conditions, current medications, and the presenting problem.* At times, the requesting physician will need your help to define what questions need to be addressed. Make sure to note the physician's name and telephone number.

3. **Is the patient aware that a psychiatric consultation has been ordered?**

   If not, ask the physician to let the patient know before you arrive.

4. **What is the patient's primary language?**

   If the patient does not speak English or another language that you can use to interview, you will want to arrange for an interpreter to meet you at the bedside.

Orders

1. Order one-to-one observation if needed. Do not let other staff members talk you out of this or convince you to delay the order once you have decided that it is warranted.

---

*It is best to have a specific question for the consultant to answer.

2. Medication orders should await examination whenever possible. If you think that urgent intramuscular (IM) or intravenous (IV) medications may be needed, ask the staff to have these available on the floor and ready for use.

■ MAJOR THREAT TO LIFE

Consultations that concern immediate threats to life are for patients who are acutely agitated and potentially harmful to themselves or others, suicidal, or refusing life-saving treatment (a decision-making–capacity consult). These issues are so important that separate chapters in this book cover each topic. Also, remember that any sudden and acute change in mental status may be a sign of an underlying life-threatening medical condition. Be alert to the patient's medical history, and do not assume that all medical conditions that might influence mental status have been ruled out.

■ COLLECTING DATA

The process of collecting data can be difficult, especially in emergency situations. Immediate interventions are often needed before a thorough evaluation can be done. When time permits, you should proceed as follows.

Chart Review

Review the patient's history systematically, noting the chief complaint; the history of present illness (HPI); the medical, surgical, and psychiatric history (including alcohol and substance abuse); the physical examination and laboratory test results; and the mental status at admission, if available. Note the circumstances of the admission (e.g., emergency transport, came in with friend or spouse), and read any social work evaluations. Then follow the patient's course in the hospital and read the events leading up to the current psychiatric consultation. Pay special attention to any recent changes in medications or medical status, notes from other consult services, and the nursing notes. Note the patient's "do not resuscitate" (DNR) status and any advance directive information, as well as the identity of the patient's emergency contact.

Information From the Treatment Team

At this point, you should have already spoken to the primary physician about the reason for the consultation. If not, try to speak with him or her now to make sure you understand the specific purpose of the consultation. If it involves refusal of treatment by a patient with a medical condition you are not familiar with, make sure that you speak with the physician about the patient's prognosis and the treatment options that the patient has, as you will need to understand this fully in order to assess the patient's ability to make a decision. Consider any countertransference issues that may be revealed in the physician's description of the situation.

Inquire from the nursing staff about the patient's behavior; attitude toward illness, staff, and visitors; compliance with medication regimen; and sleeping and eating habits. It is useful to examine countertransference issues with nonphysician staff as well. This process helps to consolidate the team approach. It is also helpful, if time allows, to personally observe the patient's interactions with the physician and with staff.

Other Sources of Information

- Check old charts whenever possible; patients may have had a psychiatric evaluation during a previous admission.
- If the patient also receives outpatient treatment at the same facility, try to obtain those records for review, and check what outpatient medications the patient was taking. Sometimes this will reveal a psychoactive medication that was discontinued upon admission of the patient to the hospital.
- Get in touch with family or friends, especially when dealing with delirious, intoxicated, or disorganized patients.
- Call the patient's regular psychiatrist or therapist, after you have the consent of the patient. Valuable data may be obtained, especially about longitudinal history and current psychotropic medications.

■ BEDSIDE

Quick Look Test

Does the patient look comfortable, distressed, agitated, or depressed? Is the patient resting in bed, in a chair, or pacing the floor? Is the staff calm or anxiously awaiting your intervention?

Establishing Rapport

After you have established that the patient is in a safe environment, it is essential that you introduce yourself and ascertain whether the requesting physician has informed the patient of the reason for your visit. If not, explain that the patient's physician has asked you to perform a psychiatric examination, and explain the reason for it. Try to make the patient as comfortable as possible in the situation before proceeding with the work-up.

The Interview

Your interview should be as focused as possible on the presenting problem and on the patient's current mental status. It is helpful to have a copy of the full mini-mental status examination so that you can give this examination to the patient when needed, as it may be an important baseline measurement for later consults.

■ CONSULT NOTE

The consultation write-up should be clear, concise, and goal directed. It is helpful to begin with a summary statement that is a one- or two-sentence description of the patient and the reason given by the treatment team for the consultation, such as, "This is a 32-year-old male patient with no known psychiatric history who was admitted for pneumonia 1 week ago. Psychiatric consult was requested because the patient has been eating very little for the past 2 days, appears depressed, and is refusing all medical tests." After this, your note should contain the following sections.

Subjective

Summarize the interview with the patient, including the patient's chief complaint and his or her own explanation of the current situation, preferably in the patient's own words. Note the patient's report or denial of relevant subjective symptoms such as hallucinations and suicidal ideation.

Objective

Include a brief summary of the patient's medical and psychiatric history, hospital course, and medical data. Then, give the mental status evaluation and results of any cognitive testing.

Assessment

In your assessment, you want to put together all the data you have gathered to reach a preliminary conclusion or differential diagnosis. As the assessment is the part of your note that will likely be read first by the treatment team, try not to use abbreviations for psychiatric terms, and clarify your thought processes briefly (in a few sentences, usually) so that the medical team understands your conclusions and recommendations. Give only the most relevant information, including positive and negative findings. List the provisional diagnosis or differential diagnoses (in descending order of likelihood) using the *Diagnostic and Statistical Manual of Mental Disorders*, 4th Edition (DSM-IV), nomenclature and the multiaxial system.

Avoid drawing premature conclusions or giving an overly simplistic explanation of the patient's behavior (e.g., writing that the patient is somatizing), which may lead to neglect of associated medical problems.

Recommendations

The usefulness of the psychiatric consultation is directly proportional to the clarity of its recommendations. Here are some points to take into account when writing your recommendations:

- Recommendations for management of acute problems should be given first. Precautionary measures for suicide such as a one-to-one watch and medications for agitation or insomnia should be implemented immediately, leaving less pressing decisions to the regular consultation team (e.g., prescribing an antidepressant).
- Give specific recommendations for tests or additional consultations that are needed to clarify the diagnosis (e.g., arterial blood gases or neurology consult), and be specific about which psychiatric or medical conditions you are considering.
- General recommendations for ongoing psychiatric care while in the hospital should be given, if appropriate. Provide your telephone number and the telephone number of the consultation service that will monitor the patient during regular work hours. If you believe the patient does need to be monitored by the consultation service, be sure to document this and state whether you will arrange for follow-up or whether the treatment team will have to arrange this.
- Finally, be very clear about your recommendations for follow-up care upon stabilization of the patient's medical condition. Is he or she a candidate for admission directly to the psychiatric unit? Will he or she need a referral to another health care facility at the time of discharge, such as an outpatient psychiatric clinic or drug and alcohol treatment program?

■ COMMUNICATING WITH THE TREATMENT TEAM

It is best to communicate your conclusions personally to the requesting physician and to the nursing staff whenever possible. This helps clarify the plan for the treatment team and resolve further questions immediately. Although the primary physician is responsible for following up on your recommendations, this promotes a team approach to the patient's management.

Whenever possible, use a consult as an opportunity to inform and educate the requesting physician and staff about the psychiatric issues related to patient care, such as countertransference issues, management of difficult patients, identification of patients who are at risk, therapeutic interventions (supportive or behavioral techniques, such as limit setting), and the use of psychotropic medications.

■ FOLLOW-UP

The consultation process is incomplete without appropriate follow-up. Be sure to inform your regular consultation-liaison team of your consultation. This is especially important for patients you see on weekends or holidays.

3 | Telephone Consultations

JULIE K. SCHULMAN

Telephone consultations are not usually a standard part of on-call work. Sometimes, however, you may be asked to handle outside telephone calls because you are the psychiatrist on call. These calls range from first contacts by people seeking psychotherapy to desperate calls by suicidal or psychotic patients. You may also get annoyance calls from people not really seeking help. Remember, there is no substitute for a face-to-face psychiatric evaluation. Over the telephone, you should focus on detecting and intervening in emergencies; otherwise, direct the caller to obtain the appropriate evaluation in person.

■ BEFORE TAKING THE CALL

Whatever the nature of the call, you should take notes on a pad or in a notebook as the telephone call proceeds. Hotlines and telephone emergency services use logbooks for this purpose. This is important both for your own accurate recollection and as a legal record of your contact with the patient.

■ IDENTIFYING DATA

You should obtain identifying data as soon as possible: name, age, telephone number, the number where the patient is calling from, and address. This may not be easy because some patients are reluctant to reveal their identities. Unless you believe that the call is hostile or manipulative, you need to proceed with an initial assessment even if the caller initially declines to identify himself or herself. Reasons for such reluctance vary. Patients who are paranoid, ashamed of their symptoms, or ambivalent about their urges to harm themselves or others may be reluctant to identify themselves. Other common reasons are concerns about confidentiality, fear of involuntary hospitalization, or fear of being forced to take medications.

If the patient refuses to provide identification and you believe the patient may pose an immediate threat to himself or herself or to others, you will need to be persistent in your attempts to identify or find the patient. Some techniques include the following.

- Piece together bits of information. Depending on your hospital, a first name alone combined with the name of the patient's doctor or the date of a recent appointment may be enough to find a computerized record. Be creative!
- You may be able to persuade some patients to let you call them back on a more private line, thereby encouraging them to reveal their phone number. A phone number alone is usually sufficient for emergency services to find them.
- Obtaining the name of the patient's therapist can be very useful. If the patient ends the call prematurely and you can reach the therapist, she or he may be able to identify the patient based on only a few details from the telephone call and can then contact the patient directly.

■ INITIAL ASSESSMENT OF RISK

Your chief concern must be the patient's immediate state of mind and dangerousness to self or others. Remember that your evaluation may be very time limited because of the patient's mental status (e.g., if the patient has taken an overdose or if the patient is paranoid and hangs up suddenly) or other emergent duties at the hospital to which you must attend. Therefore, you must work quickly. Let the patient tell you the reason for the call and describe his or her condition. Listen carefully for clues to the patient's mental status. Slurred or slowed speech may be a sign of intoxication, a medical problem, or an intentional overdose of medication.

Your questions should focus on self-harm, suicidality, and outwardly directed aggression. Be direct. Whenever suicidal or violent ideation is elicited, proceed with a detailed assessment: Does the patient have a plan and the means to enact it, such as having access to a gun? Does the patient intend to commit suicide or has he or she already made the attempt? Is there any history of suicidal or homicidal behavior? Always ask about the patient's current level of anxiety and about any recent alcohol intake or drug use. This will give you vital information about the immediate risk of suicide or violence, as both anxiety and recent use of mind-altering substances significantly increase the risk of acting on suicidal or violent impulses.

If there is a specific plan for suicide or violence or the patient has already made a suicide attempt, you need to call the police right away. Try to have someone else call the police while you keep the patient on the line. If that is not possible, tell the patient that you will call him or her back shortly, or put the person on hold, and then call the police. Stay on the line with the patient until the police arrive.

Patients who have vague suicidal ideation without a plan or intent can be reassured and encouraged to follow up with a visit to an emergency room or to their psychiatrist. Encourage the patient to call 911 if the feelings intensify. You can also suggest one of the suicide hotlines (see Appendix N).

■ OTHER INTERVENTIONS

For patients who are neither suicidal nor homicidal, you should provide brief reassurance and give an appropriate referral rather than try to treat them over the phone. The most common non-emergent phone calls are for overwhelming anxiety or panic attacks, medication questions, or questions about referral to out-patient treatment for themselves or a friend.

In cases of anxiety or depression without suicidal ideation, try to obtain information about the patient's support system. Ask with whom the patient lives, about family members or friends, and if the patient has a psychotherapist or psychiatrist. Encourage the patient to contact his or her therapist or a supportive friend or family member. If the patient has no support, you may wish to refer him or her to a hotline for further counseling or information. Some hotlines specialize in psychiatric and medical emergencies, such as the acquired immunodeficiency syndrome (AIDS), alcohol and substance abuse, and child abuse.

Avoid giving advice about medication; instead, refer patients to their prescribing physicians. For medical and legal reasons, you should never instruct a person to skip a dose or to stop taking a medication unless there is evidence of an immediate and severe potential danger to the person (e.g., a person taking lamotrigine reports a rash, or a patient who takes lithium carbonate has slurred speech and altered mental status). In these cases you will need to inform the person to come to the emergency room immediately for evaluation. Remember that you do not know the reasons the person was given the medication and that you may be held legally responsible for any future behavior by the patient that might result from discontinuing it.

If patients need immediate evaluation or inpatient treatment, encourage them to come to your emergency room or to the emergency room most accessible to them. For less urgent evaluations, you should have phone numbers available for patients to access outpatient psychiatric treatment at your facility or elsewhere.

■ ANNOYANCE CALLS

Annoyance calls are from people who may not actually be seeking help. Some of them are lonely and just want to talk.

Others have telephone paraphilias and make obscene calls. Some patients make calls threatening suicide or violence and may refuse to identify themselves or give false identification, precluding any follow-up. You should terminate such calls as soon as their nature becomes obvious (e.g., when a caller repeatedly refuses to identify himself or herself or to give an address or telephone number).

■ FOLLOW-UP

Whether or not your hospital uses a logbook, it is important to document your telephone interventions for follow-up and for legal reasons. Write down identifying data and a brief summary of the conversation, as well as your evaluation of the patient's potential dangerousness to self or others. Describe your intervention. If your patient has given you permission, call the patient's therapist to give a report of your encounter, and document this as well.

4 | Seclusion and Restraint

MARA GOLDSTEIN

This chapter defines seclusion and restraint, outlines the indications and contraindications for these procedures, and provides step-by-step guidelines for the implementation, documentation, and discontinuation of seclusion and restraint for psychiatric patients. Medication for the agitated patient, which often accompanies seclusion and restraint, is discussed in Chapter 6.

■ GENERAL PRINCIPLES

The laws, regulations, and procedures concerning the physical restraint and seclusion of patients vary from state to state and among different institutions within the same state. It is important for physicians to know the laws and policies governing the institutions in which they are working. Locked seclusion and restraint maximally restrict a patient's environment, movement, and rights. These procedures, no matter how necessary, are often frightening for patients and are experienced as degrading. Seclusion and restraint should be used with tact and discretion in a limited number of situations and for therapeutic reasons only.

■ LITERATURE REVIEW

A literature review on the topic of seclusion and restraint led Fisher[1] to reach the following conclusions concerning the risks and benefits of these interventions:

- Seclusion and restraint are basically efficacious in preventing injury and reducing agitation.
- It is nearly impossible to operate a program for severely symptomatic individuals without some form of seclusion or physical or mechanical restraint.
- Restraint and seclusion may have deleterious physical and psychologic effects on patients and staff.
- Local nonclinical factors, such as cultural biases, staff role perceptions, and the attitude of hospital administration, have a substantial influence on rates of restraint and seclusion.
- Training in the prediction and prevention of violence, in self-defense, and in the implementation of restraint and/or

seclusion is valuable in reducing the rates and untoward effects of these procedures.

■ DEFINITIONS

1. Seclusion
   a. Open seclusion: The therapeutic isolation of a patient. Methods of open seclusion include quiet time alone in a patient's room, in an unlocked time-out room, or in a partitioned area. Open seclusion represents the least restrictive form of seclusion. Most regulations referring to seclusion relate specifically to locked seclusion only.
   b. Locked seclusion: The therapeutic isolation of a patient in a locked room designed specifically for the purpose of confining an agitated individual.
2. Restraint: A confining apparatus commonly composed of leather or canvas. When properly applied, restraints maximally restrict physical movement without threatening the integrity of the limb or body part being restrained. Restraint configurations include
   a. Bilateral wristlets and anklets; also known as four-point restraint
   b. Camisole controlling the upper half of the body with or without bilateral anklets
   c. Chest strap with either of the above
   d. Whole-body restraints, such as safety suits, which contain the patient's entire body with the exception of the head

■ INDICATIONS AND CONTRAINDICATIONS

Indications

- Prevention of imminent harm to the patient or to others when other means are ineffective
- Prevention of substantial damage to the physical environment

Indications for seclusion **without** physical restraint include

- Decreasing stimulation for an agitated, potentially violent patient
- Fulfilling a patient's request in appropriate circumstances, such as self-awareness of poor impulse control or low frustration tolerance

Contraindications

- For the convenience or comfort of staff
- To punish a patient

Absolute contraindications specific to seclusion include
- The acutely suicidal patient (without constant observation)
- The patient with unstable medical status
- The delirious or otherwise neurologically impaired patient whose clinical status may decline when stimulation is reduced
- The restrained patient who cannot be adequately monitored for aspiration or circulatory impairment

Relative contraindications specific to seclusion include
- The self-mutilating patient (without constant observation)
- The patient with a seizure disorder
- The hyperactive patient at risk for exhaustion
- The developmentally disabled patient (see below)

■ SPECIAL CONSIDERATIONS

Developmental Disabilities

Patients with documented developmental disabilities are at higher risk for injury during restraint and seclusion procedures and during the period of the restraint and/or seclusion. Such patients may have underlying physical anomalies, particularly craniofacial and cardiac, that can further endanger their safety during restraint and seclusion procedures. Developmentally disabled persons may not be able to understand why such interventions have been imposed and may not be able to communicate their discomfort while in restraints or while being secluded.

Children

Mechanical restraint and locked seclusion are not generally used for young or small children. A technique called *therapeutic holding* is often employed to help control agitated and dangerous children. This typically entails hugging a child from behind, whereby his or her arms are held securely to each side. This technique requires training, and the physician on call should be familiar with the procedures used at his or her facility.

Victims of Abuse

Patients with a personal history of abuse may experience restraints and locked seclusion as especially traumatic, particularly if some aspect of their initial traumatic event is re-created during the sequence of the locked seclusion or restraint procedure. Staff members should be sensitive to issues pertaining to patients who are victims of abuse.

■ PHYSICIAN RESPONSE

Seclusion and restraint are frequently initiated on an emergent basis by nurses or other trained staff on the psychiatric ward. In such cases, continuation of the seclusion or restraint will require a physician's assessment, documentation, and written order. The expectation is that the physician on call will be contacted immediately to complete these tasks. Again, it is important for physicians to be familiar with the guidelines of each facility where they will be on call regarding the time parameters for physician notification and response. Most agencies have a time limit beyond which delays must be explained in the documentation. When there are large geographic distances between sites, the physician may want to discuss this issue with a hospital administrator.

If the physician arrives on the scene before initiation of the procedure, he or she should participate in the coordination and preparation of the intervention team as described below.

■ PROCEDURE FOR LOCKED SECLUSION AND RESTRAINT

Locked seclusion and/or restraint procedures are undertaken after the failure of the patient to accept oral medication and/or open seclusion. Subduing a dangerous individual should be a team effort involving a sufficient number of adequately trained professionals such as nurses, physicians, mental health technicians, and often security personnel. It is not unusual for the entire procedure to take place in the absence of a physician, particularly after regular working hours. The physician on call must be notified immediately so that he or she may go to the area with the patient as quickly as possible.

Team

The team is ideally made up of at least eight trained staff members. One team leader is designated. The team leader instructs the others throughout the procedure while maintaining truthful and reassuring dialogue with the patient. A staff member with whom the patient is more familiar may be perceived by the patient as more comforting and therefore may be a good choice for the team leader.

One team member is assigned to each of the patient's limbs, and a fifth is assigned to protect and control the patient's head. One team member (a nurse) should be assigned to provide the necessary medications. The exact number of staff required for the procedure depends on individual factors such as patient size and level of agitation. All of the assignment decisions should be made before the procedure is implemented.

Once a leader has been chosen, he or she should assign tasks among the remaining staff. An individual who is too agitated and volatile to comply with less restrictive alternatives will generally resist seclusion or restraints. The presence of a large team as well as backup such as hospital security or police is referred to as a "show of force." This is often helpful in encouraging compliance. Some facilities require the presence of hospital security or police before the initiation of seclusion and restraint procedures, although whether such persons may participate in the actual procedure varies among facilities. Sometimes the team decides on a prearranged signal to begin the procedure, such as an extended head nod. The leader may use this signal if necessary to indicate the initiation of physical force in order to achieve seclusion or restraint.

Logistics

Before the patient is approached, the environment must be cleared of extraneous people and physical hazards. A team member should prepare a bed or stretcher suitable to accommodate mechanical restraints, with restraints on standby. Injectible medication should be drawn and made available as indicated. To maximize safety, all staff involved should remove any ties, scarves, dangling jewelry, and similar items and wear latex gloves. Face masks for the team members, particularly the one assigned to the patient's head, may be useful in the event the patient starts spitting.

Approach

When approaching the patient, the team members should gather around the leader and calmly present themselves in a confident yet caring, nonthreatening, nonprovocative manner. The leader should provide the patient with a simple explanation of why seclusion or restraint is required. Only the leader should be speaking to the patient at this time. The patient should be given the option to voluntarily comply with the least restrictive measure clinically appropriate to the situation. The patient should be allowed several seconds in order to follow directions.

Negotiating with the patient at this point is ill-advised. Doing so may lead to further escalation and violence.

Implementation

If the patient does not comply, the leader should give the prearranged signal, indicating that the team will proceed with the use of force to achieve seclusion or restraint. Four team members should then take hold of and control each limb previously assigned. The patient should then be carefully brought to the ground, usually in a supine position, on a padded surface if available. The head should be controlled, using caution to avoid skull, neck, and facial injuries while attempting to protect staff from biting or spitting. Special attention to safety is imperative, particularly when dealing with physically challenged, elderly, pregnant, and developmentally disabled patients, who may be more vulnerable to injury in the process.

The patient should then be transferred to the seclusion room or the area where restraints are applied. Head, trunk, and extended legs are lifted simultaneously on the count of the team leader. Extended arms are held securely to the sides of the patient as he or she is moved and placed on a bed or stretcher. The head is placed toward the seclusion room door.

Intramuscular medication should be injected at the point of maximal immobilization. This often occurs during the period between the take-down and the application of restraints.

If the patient has been brought to the seclusion room without the application of restraints, team members should release the limbs sequentially after the administration of intramuscular medication, as indicated. The staff members should be careful to assess the patient's status as each limb is released and should be careful to keep an eye on the patient as they leave the seclusion room.

Of note, most staff injuries related to patient care occur during the implementation of seclusion and restraint. The incidence of these injuries can be decreased with improved training programs for staff in the area of violence prediction, violence assessment, restraint and seclusion procedures, and self-defense.

Debriefing

A debriefing session should follow as soon as possible after the procedure. This involves a gathering of all the staff involved in the seclusion and/or restraint procedure for the purpose of discussing the events. Debriefings serve several functions:

- Analyze and critique the intervention process
- Discuss feelings and concerns about the incident
- Solidify the cohesion of the team
- Prevent future misuse of imposed restrictions. This includes

either implementing seclusion and restraint when not appropriate or avoiding these modalities when they are indicated
- Allow for team assessment in the event of a staff injury

Patient

Although it is the safety of the patient, other patients, and the staff that is of utmost importance, the physician and the staff should proceed with as much care and compassion as possible. What is accurately perceived as necessary by the staff may be perceived as embarrassing, humiliating, and frightening for the patient, even when he or she believes the intervention to be necessary.[1] Staff should help patients to discuss the experience. A dialogue with the patient should begin while he or she is still in restraints. It is also important to be prepared to discuss the intervention with other patients on the ward who will likely react differently according to their own personal histories with restraints and seclusion. Those patients who have never been restrained or secluded often feel safer seeing a potentially violent patient removed from the open space of the ward. Those who have been restrained or secluded in the past may feel angry when they see another patient undergoing a similar procedure.

■ DOCUMENTATION

Seclusion and restraint procedures command the same intensity of charting as do other emergency patient care situations. Although documentation may appear to be lengthy and cumbersome, it is designed to protect patients from potential misuse.

Hospital Forms

Hospitals frequently stock preprinted mandatory seclusion and restraint forms, or log sheets, which may fulfill the institution's initial charting obligations. On-call physicians should verify whether such a form exists in the facility in which they are working as well as whether a separate progress note is required. The permanent nursing staff is an excellent resource and may be able to help the physician become familiar with the forms and logs.

Note

A progress note with the physician's observations is extremely important even if it is not required. This note should be placed in the patient's regular unit chart. The following information should be included in the documentation of a seclusion or restraint procedure, regardless of the charting format:

- The patient's last name and first name
- Chart or medical record number
- Date and time of incident
- The time of the physician's arrival on the scene
- Justification for a late arrival on the scene if it is longer than the required time after notification; the nursing staff is required to note the time of physician notification, and it is wise for the physician to do so as well
- The precipitating event, in a detailed fashion, specifying dangerous behavior
- Failure of the patient to respond to less restrictive measures such as verbal redirection and/or offers of oral medication
- The restrictive measures implemented (e.g., locked seclusion, four-point leather restraints)
- Clinical justification for these measures, which includes pertinent findings on mental status examination and specific behavior
- Length of time the restriction will be imposed; this must include the starting and ending times
- Behavioral goals to be met by the patient in order to have the restriction lifted, such as the ability to stay in an open room calmly for 20 minutes; this must also be verbalized to the patient
- Patient response to the procedure; again, an attempt should be made to continue a dialogue with the patient while in restraint or seclusion
- The printed name and signature of the physician

It is also useful to document that the patient and his or her environment have been checked and that potentially dangerous materials have been removed.

Written Order

The written order for seclusion or restraint must include the date and time the restriction was imposed, as well as the time it will be lifted. Phrases such as "2 hours" are not considered sufficiently specific. Indicate exactly the type of restriction to be implemented and the justification for its use (e.g., for assaultive or self-injurious behavior). Some states require release criteria to be included in the written order. Seclusion and restraints may never be ordered on an as-needed (PRN) basis.

■ CONTINUATION AND DISCONTINUATION OF RESTRICTIONS

Many jurisdictions require that every patient in locked seclusion or restraints should be on one-to-one observation. These are patients for whom the maximally restrictive setting has been imposed for safety reasons. While this may not be the standard of practice in every institution across the country, it remains within the physician's purview to order one-to-one observation.

Periodic progress notes should include a mental status examination; references to the patient's physical stability, including vital signs and ability to tolerate restraints; and the patient's progress toward meeting the expectations that will facilitate the lifting of restrictions. Restrictions may be removed once a secluded or restrained patient has fulfilled pre-established criteria and appears clinically stable such that he or she no longer presents a threat to self, others, or the environment.

An individual in locked seclusion or restraints should gradually have restrictions lifted contingent on the ability to maintain calmness and safety. The suggested procedure for ending seclusion is to open the seclusion room door for 15 to 30 minutes while asking the patient to stay inside.

■ SAFETY WARNINGS

Leaving only one extremity in restraint can lead to avoidable patient injury and is not permissible in many jurisdictions. Restraints should be periodically checked by nursing staff.

Some situations involving mechanical restraints or seclusion affect the patient's temperature regulation. This can add to the effects of antipsychotic medications on temperature regulation, potentially leading to hyperthermia or neuroleptic malignant syndrome.

Reference

1. Fisher WA: Seclusion and restraint: a review of the literature. Am J Psychiatry 1994;151(11):1584–1591.

5 | Assessment of Competency and Other Legal Issues

MARA GOLDSTEIN

This chapter discusses issues of competency, decisional capacity, and informed consent as well as the voluntary and involuntary treatment of psychiatric patients. The physician should be familiar with the laws, statutes, and institutional policies governing the legal aspects of psychiatry in the jurisdiction in which he or she is practicing.

■ DEFINITIONS

Competency

Competency is a legal term that refers to the legal capacity of an adult to perform a specific function. Competency can be formally determined only by a judge. Any patient who has not been found incompetent via legal proceedings is, by legal definition, a competent individual. A competent individual, however, may lack "decisional capacity" with respect to certain medical interventions. In a clinical setting competency and decisional capacity are used synonymously, but they are not the same. Psychiatrists do not make the final legal determinations about competency.

Decisional capacity is a clinical term that describes a person's functional ability to make informed decisions about treatment. Decisional capacity is also task specific and can change over the course of illness. It can be affected by a person's response to stress, by the medications that he or she is receiving, or by an underlying and potentially treatable mental illness. The assessment of decisional capacity can be a time-consuming task, requiring the analysis and integration of ethical, legal, and clinical elements.

Informed consent refers to the process by which patients knowingly and willingly agree to a specific treatment. To agree knowingly to a treatment, a patient must be provided with all relevant information regarding his or her condition, including the risks and benefits of the various procedures and treatments available as well as the risk of no treatment at all. To be able to provide informed consent, a patient must be able to communicate each of the following: a choice about the treatment, an understanding of the relevant information, an appreciation of the situation as it pertains to his or her life, and evidence of a rational thought process (see below). Patients must make their decisions freely and voluntarily.

■ ROLE OF THE CONSULTING PSYCHIATRIST ON NONPSYCHIATRIC SERVICES

Although consulting psychiatrists cannot adjudicate competency, they can evaluate the patient's mental capacity to give informed consent or to give an informed refusal and to participate in the decision-making process regarding the treatment option in question. The following is a set of screening questions to ask when the treating physician initiates a request for psychiatric consultation:

- What is the specific procedure or treatment at hand?
- Has the physician attempted to obtain informed consent? What exactly was the patient told about the procedure?
- What is the urgency with which the procedure must be done?
- Is the patient suffering from a medical condition that may be impairing his or her cognition?
- What medications is the patient taking?
- Has the physician or any other staff member noted abnormalities in the mental status of the patient?
- Does the patient have a legal guardian?
- Who is the next of kin, and is there a health care proxy?
- Does the patient have a living will or advanced directives?
- What is the physician's and other health professionals' sense of the patient's decisional capacity?

The treating physician and other health professionals need to be informed that the psychiatric assessment will be valid only for the procedure for which it was requested and for the time period in which the evaluation was performed.

■ ASSESSMENT

The assessment of the patient should begin with a thorough history. This includes a review of the patient's chart, laboratory test results, and medications. The consulting psychiatrist should perform a detailed mental status examination as well as assess for the presence of any psychiatric disorder. When illnesses such as depression, delirium, psychosis, and pseudodementia are present, lack of decisional capacity may be temporary. In some cases, however, the urgency of the treatment and the risk of delay may not allow time for the physician to fully treat the underlying illness.

The assessment of judgment is specific to the task at hand. The physician should consider the patient's general capacity to grasp the nature of the situation, to become engaged in the decision-making process, and to act on his or her own behalf. The following is a list of questions that can help in assessing the patient's understanding and preference[1]:

- What is the patient's understanding of the medical problem?
- What is the patient's understanding of the physician's recommendations?
- What is the patient's understanding of the physician's rationale?
- What is the patient's choice?
- What is the patient's rationale for the choice?
- What does the patient anticipate as the consequences of exercising his or her choice?
- What is the patient's understanding of the risks and benefits of the recommended treatment? Of alternative treatments? Of no treatment?

According to Appelbaum and Grisso,[2] the legal standards for competence include the four skills of communicating a choice, understanding relevant information, appreciating the current situation and its consequences, and manipulating information rationally. This ability may be affected by an impairment of consciousness, a thought disorder, or a disruption in short-term memory.

- **Communicating a choice**: The patient must be able to communicate a preference with respect to his or her care. This concept requires that the patient be able to maintain choices long enough for them to be implemented.
- **Understanding relevant information**: The patient must be able to receive and retain the information that is provided. The patient should be able to describe the details of the procedure, why it is necessary, what the risks and benefits are, and when it is likely to take place.
- **Appreciating the situation and its consequences**: Appreciation of the situation implies that the patient can assess, according to his or her own values, the impact of the situation at hand. To appreciate the situation and its consequences, the patient must be able to grasp what the risks and benefits mean to him or her, including likely outcomes, and the potentials for pain and suffering both with and without treatment. The patient should be able to express an appreciation of the impact of the decision on his or her quality of life. Depression, for example, may impair one's capacity for appreciation.
- **Manipulating information rationally**: The patient must be able to use logical thought processes to compare the benefits and risks of various treatment options. It is the process of weighing pros and cons. Rational manipulation involves the ability to reach conclusions logically consistent with the starting premise.

As the consequences of a patient's decision to consent to or refuse treatment become more serious, the criteria for assessing competency should become more stringent. This is also known as the *sliding scale* or the *risk-benefit model*. The degree to which the criteria for decisional capacity are applied often depends on the risk that the patient assumes with his or her decision. The more risk assumed by the patient's decision, the more stringently applied the criteria will be in the assessment. For example, the above criteria may be less stringently applied in the assessment of a patient refusing to have vital signs taken versus a patient refusing life-saving cardiac catheterization.

■ COMMUNICATING FINDINGS

Once the assessment has been made, the consulting psychiatrist should discuss his or her findings with the team or treating physician. If a patient is believed to lack decisional capacity in a certain situation, then it is the duty of the team to proceed to the next level of obtaining consent. Does the patient have a health care proxy? Does the patient have a legal or medical guardian? Is there a living will? Who is the next of kin? What power does the hospital have to grant administrative consent?

The next step for the team will depend on the laws of the state and the policies and procedures of the facility in which the patient is being treated, as well as the urgency with which the intervention or procedure in question must be implemented. Administrative consultation is likely to be needed at this point. In the event of a medical emergency, however, when delay for consultation of any kind is acutely dangerous, informed consent is assumed until the state of emergency has passed. It is also helpful for the treating team to discuss cases in which administrative consent is required with the hospital's risk management or legal department.

■ ADMISSION OF PATIENTS TO A PSYCHIATRIC FACILITY

There are four basic types of admission to a general civil hospital. Each state may have different laws governing the mechanisms of admission, with different hospitals across the state using one or more of these mechanisms. Psychiatrists should be aware of the laws governing the admission of psychiatric patients within their state as well as the policies of the various institutions in which they practice.

- **Informal admission**: Informal admission is the same as a general hospital admission. The patient is free to enter and leave at will, as there is an absence of any formal legal status. Most hospitals do not use this mechanism of admission.
- **Voluntary admission**: A competent person seeking psychiatric care may apply in writing for admission to most psychiatric facilities. The patient requires examination by a physician or mental health professional. Once admitted voluntarily, a patient may or may not be allowed to leave the hospital at will. The amount of time a voluntary patient can be detained against his or her will in order to assess his or her safety varies from state to state. If release is unsafe, the team may go to court for an involuntary civil commitment hearing. This procedure is explained to the patient through a formal notice of status and rights when he or she signs in to the hospital.
- **Emergency admission**: In the case of the emergency admission, the patient is in need of immediate hospitalization but is unable or unwilling to make this decision for himself or herself. Such patients may be too disturbed to make a decision regarding their own care and are deemed a danger to themselves or others outside the hospital. This type of admission status is time limited, and the time frame for the patient to remain at this status is usually shorter than that of an involuntary admission.
- **Involuntary admission**: This type of admission is appropriate for patients who are mentally ill and a danger to themselves or others, or who cannot care for themselves secondary to a mental illness, and are unable or unwilling to consent to immediate hospitalization. A physician, friend, relative, or, in some jurisdictions, a community agency director may submit an application for admission to the courts. The patient may be retained only until a court hearing yields a decision on further retention or release. The patient must have access to legal counsel and must be provided with a formal notice of status and rights. A judge can release the patient at any time if it is determined that the commitment criteria are not met. This type of admission is time limited as well.

■ INVOLUNTARY TREATMENT OF PSYCHIATRIC PATIENTS

Psychiatric patients have a right to refuse treatment even if they have been hospitalized against their will. This can be overridden only under special circumstances. In most jurisdictions, nonemergency forced treatment requires an administrative or judicial hearing. Nearly all states allow for exceptions when emergency circumstances arise. An emergency is said to exist when a patient suffering from a mental illness poses an imminent risk of bodily harm to self or to others in the treatment setting. Forced treatment to prevent such harm is permitted when it represents the least restrictive method of intervention in an emergency. A physician who orders a treatment to be administered against the wishes of a patient should carefully document his or her findings of a direct examination of the patient, the basis for the decision, and how the treatment is the least restrictive alternative to maintain safety.

■ DISCHARGE

The physician on call may be asked to discharge a patient against the patient's wishes. These circumstances include when a patient knowingly violates a rule, such as smuggling drugs or alcohol into the hospital, or has been restored to health but refuses to leave. A similar situation arises when a patient is seeking psychiatric admission but the physician on call does not believe that an admission is necessary or appropriate. In these situations, it is important to document the reasons why hospitalization, or continued hospitalization, is being refused. Documentation of the situation should be thorough, and it should include the opinions of consultants and other professionals whenever possible. The patient should be provided with other options for care such as a referral to a more appropriate treatment facility. The patient should know that he or she can return for re-evaluation, as a patient cannot be refused care in an emergency.

The on-call physician is often asked to evaluate patients requesting discharge from medical or psychiatric settings who cannot be safely discharged owing to acute illness. In these cases, the physician will need to evaluate the patient's decisional capacity to leave the hospital using the guidelines outlined earlier in this chapter. If the patient is competent, he or she may still require further involuntary detention if there is an immediate risk to the safety of the patient or to others as a result of an underlying mental illness. Making these decisions involves knowing the laws in the areas in which the physician is practicing.

■ CONFIDENTIALITY

Confidentiality is the obligation of the physician not to share information provided by the patient unless the patient gives permission to do so. Exceptions to confidentiality include
- Emergency situations for urgent interventions
- Mandated reporting of child abuse or suspected child abuse

- Reportable diseases
- Firearm and knife wounds
- Duties to inform third parties

Tarasoff (*Tarasoff* v. *Regents of the University of California*) and related "duty to warn" court cases have established in many jurisdictions that a physician has the duty to warn or to protect potential victims. The psychiatrist may have to notify the police and/or the potential victim of danger threatened by a patient who is being released or has left a facility without permission. The American Psychiatric Association guidelines suggest that confidentiality may be broken when a patient is likely to commit suicide or murder and can be stopped only by notification of police. Confidentiality may also be broken when a person may endanger the lives of others owing to impairment, such as an impaired pilot or bus driver.

References

1. Kaplan KH, Price M: The clinician's role in competency evaluations. Gen Hosp Psychiatry 1989;11:397–403.
2. Appelbaum PS, Grisso T: Assessing patients' capacities to consent to treatment. N Engl J Med 1988;319(25):1635–1638.

6 | The Difficult Patient

MICHELLE E. MONTEMAYOR

A common request a psychiatric physician receives is to assess a difficult patient. Often the situation is a complex one in which the staff, the patient, and the patient's family may all contribute to the problematic behavior expressed by the patient. Such patients are characterized as manipulative, entitled, demanding, needy, verbally inappropriate, or abusive. The patient may feel that ward rules are too constricting or that his or her needs are not taken seriously by the staff. Staff members often feel frustrated when patients do not follow rules intended for safety or make trivial demands when more urgent patient care is at stake. Managing such episodes can be especially challenging at night, when wards have limited personnel to devote to the problem.

■ PHONE CALL

Questions

1. **What is the acuity of the situation?**
   - Is the patient verbally or physically assaultive to other patients or staff members? If so, is the patient able to respond to verbal redirection?
   - Has oral as-needed (PRN) medication been offered?
   - Is one-to-one staff supervision necessary?
   - If the patient is unable or unwilling to respond verbally, has hospital security been called to assist in bringing the patient under control by administration of intramuscular PRN medication and/or seclusion and restraints?
2. **Once the potential dangerousness is managed, attempt to characterize the cause(s) and duration of the trouble.**
   - What is the source of the patient's distress?
   - Is the current problem associated with the patient's ongoing behavior, or is this an isolated incident?
   - Are other patients or family members involved?
   - Is the ward milieu being disrupted?
   - Is the patient attempting to leave the hospital against medical advice?

3. **What efforts have been made to attend to the problem thus far?**
   - Has any staff member attempted to discuss the issue with the patient?
   - Has the patient been reminded of the hospital rules that he or she agreed to as a condition for admission?
   - Is there a consistent plan for dealing with the consequences of difficult patient behavior with appropriate limit setting?

Orders

1. When the patient is endangering himself or herself or others, ask the nurse to call hospital security. In most cases, a show of force (i.e., arrival of several members of the security team) is enough to persuade the patient to respond to verbal redirection before the psychiatrist's arrival.
2. Ask the nurse to make restraints and PRN intramuscular medication available. If possible, have staff hold off on these measures until you have had a chance to evaluate the situation.

Inform RN

If the patient is out of control, immediate response is indicated. For less acute situations, it is important to remember that these are among the most frustrating situations for staff members. Communicate your sincere desire to help staff deal with the problem in a timely fashion. An ongoing problem with a difficult patient is often perceived as an urgent problem for overburdened staff members. Give a realistic estimate of your time of arrival to the floor, and ascertain if this is acceptable to staff. Verbal support for staff efforts alleviates some of the anxiety generated by a difficult patient and may help you to negotiate the time required to deal with more acute problems on a busy service.

■ ELEVATOR THOUGHTS

Difficult patients are usually trying to get attention or emotional support from staff members and may make impossible demands. Anything from lack of manners to severe Axis I, II, or III pathology may contribute to such behavior. If a patient feels abandoned or neglected, his or her behavior may be significant for neediness, entitled demands, low frustration tolerance and anger, impulsiveness, and rule breaking.
   - Fearfulness is often expressed with somatization, irritability, or paranoia. If the patient is psychotic, he or she may not be

organized enough to communicate the nature of his or her problem. Alternatively, panic and/or a sense of doom may be symptoms of a serious medical condition (e.g., myocardial infarction or asthma attack).

- The patient may have undiagnosed, undertreated, or newly treated mania, depression, or psychosis manifesting as anger, impatience, neediness, or recklessness.
- The patient may be having difficulty with pain, sleep, appetite, or bowel movements. Medication side effects are possible. Ongoing illicit drug or alcohol use and/or withdrawal may be involved.
- The patient may be having interpersonal difficulty with family or other patients and expressing it toward staff. Primitive attempts to get help are often viewed as manipulative gestures by staff. Anger or scorn directed toward the patient only makes the patient feel more marginalized and may escalate his or her acting out.

Typically, the patient has poor interpersonal skills and is labeled a "troublemaker." Once this title is bestowed, even the most innocent of requests can be met with significant staff disdain. Here, your attitude can make a difference.

Periodically, the daytime staff "promises" that the patient will get a particular test, treatment, or service that cannot be provided during the night shift; the patient having little control over his or her hospital regimen can feel neglected or abused or misunderstood and take his or her frustration out on night staff.

Identifying sources of the patient's distress and taking steps to ameliorate it will put the patient at ease. Once the patient is in a more receptive mood, more appropriate ways to ask for staff help can be discussed. Often, tactful review of the patient's concerns with staff will enlist the patient's help in coming up with a meaningful solution to the problem at hand.

■ MAJOR THREAT TO LIFE

- Unrecognized medical or psychiatric problem

  Withdrawal from alcohol or illicit drugs and medical or psychiatric conditions may first come to attention in the context of the "difficult patient." Although other staff may minimize the signs and symptoms of a possible medical or psychiatric illness, you should take such signs as seriously as you would when dealing with other patients.

- Physical injury

  Difficult patients often elicit strong emotions from the staff. It is hard to remember that a patient is frightened, in pain, or feeling abandoned when he or she is agitated and threatening. Once a staff member has been injured or insulted, objectivity can be very difficult to maintain. Check your own tone of voice and attitude, and do all you can to remain neutral.

If a patient is threatening to harm himself or herself or staff, institute one-to-one observation of the patient. Take necessary measures to ensure safety. Medication, seclusion, and/or restraint may be involved. It is important to instruct the patient on the level of behavioral control that must be exhibited before discontinuation of orders instituted to ensure the patient's safety.

■ BEDSIDE

Quick Look Test

As the physician called to assess the problem, you can help neutralize a potentially violent situation. Remain as calm as possible. Speak slowly and softly, and be as respectful as possible to all parties involved.

As you enter the ward, quickly assess the emotional tone of the atmosphere. If the staff and patients are calm, listen attentively to everyone's concerns. Make your best effort to be nonjudgmental; do not take sides—remain neutral. In this scenario, reinforcement of ward rules, additional medication, or a simple supportive plan may be all that is necessary. Once the problem is delineated and the plan is set, give all parties positive feedback.

When you are met with an emotionally charged atmosphere, calm discussion may not be an option. You may have to order PRN medication, seclusion, and/or restraint and then wait for everyone to settle down before discussing the situation. Safety takes precedence over any other concern.

Frequently, the situation is between the two extremes described above. The patient and staff member(s) are exasperated with each other, and you are being asked to settle the dispute. When you deal with this type of scenario, it is important to be aware of unconscious issues. Patients may express intense rage or dependent needs in ways that are overwhelming to staff. Some patients are particularly adroit at fostering distrust among hospital colleagues or capitalizing on underlying staff disputes. One staff member may be pitted against another, destabilizing the ward milieu. Alternatively, the patient may come to be viewed as "intolerable" or "hateful." In such situations, your neutrality is necessary to provide a calm, stable atmosphere for conflict resolution.

■ MANAGEMENT

It is important to remember that most problems that manifest with respect to the difficult patient are complex and ongoing. In most cases, you will not be able to solve the problem. Your task is to furnish temporizing measures that will permit the staff to continue to care for the patient in the least restrictive manner and in the safest possible environment. In addition, it is your responsibility to document clearly and concisely in your chart notes the events that have transpired. Make sure to give a detailed account of your intervention and the limit of its success. If warranted, contact the primary physician and give verbal sign-out in the morning. Such professional courtesy is greatly appreciated by your colleagues.

The best way to deal with the difficult patient is to elicit a compromise that will allow both staff and the patient to achieve some element of their desired result. The patient may demand to leave the hospital or to smoke cigarettes, both of which may be impossible requests of the covering physician. Calm but firm reiteration of hospital rules is necessary. You may choose to offer the edgy patient experiencing nicotine withdrawal a snack or sedative medication. You may also indicate in your note that a nicotine patch may be worth the consideration of the primary physician in the morning. If the patient is demanding to leave the hospital, try to find out what precipitated this decision. If possible, address it. Often, the complaint is simple: "My roommate is snoring; I can't sleep here; I want to sleep at home." A simple room reassignment or allowing the patient to sleep in an open common room may help him or her to remain in the hospital without distress. If the particular problem cannot be addressed immediately, furnish the patient with information that will allow him or her to contact the patient representative, legal service, or ombudsman office in the morning.

If a patient is on a detoxification protocol and is requesting additional medication, assess vital signs and physical symptoms of withdrawal. In many instances, additional or alternative medications are justified. Make sure that the requested medication does not contradict the primary physician's treatment plan. If the medication is not in keeping with the plan, try to offer another medication that will address the patient's symptoms. If the distressed patient is difficult to calm, a single small dose of an atypical antipsychotic may be preferable to a benzodiazepine to provide sedation and anxiolytic effects without the addictive properties.

■ REMEMBER

When dealing with situations generated by the difficult patient, focus on definition of the issue and the causes and conditions by which it arose. Both the patient and the staff have concerns that will need to be addressed. Listen as nonjudgmentally as possible. Be supportive and compliment positive efforts where they exist. Enlist the help of the patient and the staff to characterize the problem and to work toward its immediate solution. Set limits where necessary in a firm, matter-of-fact manner. Acknowledge that the solution may not be optimal. In the morning, further options may be explored by the primary physician and staff.

7 | The Emergency Evaluation of Children and Adolescents

AVA ALBRECHT
MARK KRUSHELNYCKY

The on-call psychiatrist may be consulted to evaluate a child or adolescent in the emergency room, on a medical floor, or on an inpatient unit. Depending on the site, the consultation may be for an initial evaluation, for management of an acutely agitated patient, or for evaluation of a newly emergent psychiatric or medical condition.

The evaluation of children and adolescents differs from that of adults in several ways. A comprehensive evaluation requires information about family, school, and social relationships in order to evaluate the overall functioning of the patient. This often requires the involvement of other sources of information, including parents or legal guardians, social workers, teachers, and other professionals or organizations that may be involved in the care of the patient. Management of the acutely agitated child or adolescent should be as conservative as possible, and any concerns about medical issues that arise on the inpatient psychiatric unit should be addressed with the pediatrician on call.

■ PHONE CALL

The call to you may be as ambiguous as "We have a child for you to evaluate." As with other calls for a consultation, clarify the reason for the consultation.

Questions

1. Where is the patient?
2. What is the age of the patient?
3. Who brought the patient to the hospital, and why?
4. Has the patient had a physical examination? If so, are there any abnormalities?
5. Does the patient take medications? If so, what?
6. Has the patient abused drugs or alcohol?
7. Does the patient require seclusion or one-to-one observation?

Orders/Inform RN

1. Request that the patient be searched for weapons and other instruments that may cause injury. This should especially be considered for those with a history of carrying weapons.
2. Have the patient placed in a room where he or she will be safe. This may require one-to-one observation, especially if the patient is assaultive, aggressive, suicidal, or an elopement risk. Consider the layout of the area in which the patient will be waiting for evaluation to make sure that it is adequate for the safety of the patient.
3. Request that any accompanying adults wait until you can speak with them.

Let the RN know when you will evaluate the patient. If medical clearance is not yet complete, you may ask that it be done before your evaluation. Order old records.

■ ELEVATOR THOUGHTS

Whom will you interview first?

Generally, parents are interviewed first when the patient is a child. When an adolescent is the patient, he or she is interviewed first.

For which conditions are children and adolescents brought to the emergency room?

Most children are brought for evaluation of suicidal ideation, aggression, inability of parents or teachers to control behavior, risk-taking behavior, physical abuse, or bizarre behaviors. Some children are brought in because the family needs crisis intervention.

What conditions and behaviors are emergencies that require hospitalization?

A patient who attempts to harm himself or herself or others probably requires hospitalization. Children who are extremely impulsive, live in an abusive environment, or are psychotic are at high risk for engaging in harmful behaviors and may also require hospitalization.

Is the adult accompanying the patient the legal guardian? If not, who is?

It is important to attempt to establish contact with the patient's legal guardian. He or she will need to be informed about the results of the evaluation and to be involved in treatment decisions.

For a chief complaint of suicidal ideation, consider
- Mood disorders
- Psychosis

- Intoxication or substance abuse
- Attention-seeking or manipulative behavior
- Physical or sexual abuse

For a complaint of aggression or homicidal ideation, consider
- Behavioral disorders, such as conduct disorder and attention-deficit/hyperactivity disorder (ADHD)
- Intoxication or substance abuse
- Psychosis
- Mental retardation and autism
- Physical or sexual abuse

Again, remember to rule out other medical and metabolic causes for the behaviors, including, for example, temporal lobe epilepsy and infection.

■ MAJOR THREAT TO LIFE

Suicidal and homicidal ideation and self-injurious behavior require that the patient be kept in a safe environment. To complete a comprehensive evaluation, both you and the patient must be in a safe place. This is necessary to protect you, the patient, anyone accompanying the patient, and others in the area.

■ BEDSIDE

Selective History and Chart Review

The evaluation of children and adolescents should be a comprehensive evaluation. It must include the following:
- Chief complaint
- History of present illness (HPI), including recent psychosocial stressors
- Past psychiatric history
- Medications and compliance
- Habits, including specific types of alcohol and recreational drugs used, such as marijuana, cocaine, crack, lysergic acid diethylamide (LSD), heroin, "Ecstasy" (methylenedioxymethamphetamine), stimulants, inhalants, over-the-counter medications, "natural" medications, diet supplements, and abuse of prescription medications
- Birth and developmental history
- Social history, including current level of functioning with family, peers, school, relationships, and stressors in all spheres
- Family history
- Mental status examination
- Physical examination, including toxicology screen, pregnancy test, and serum levels for medications

You must ask the patient and a reliable informant about certain potentially dangerous behaviors. These serious behaviors and

symptoms include setting fires, carrying weapons, suicidal ideation, homicidal ideation, psychosis, molesting others, truancy,
and a history of arrest. Ask about these behaviors even if the
chief complaint seems completely unrelated. It may also be important to ask about sexual activity, eating habits, and self-injurious behaviors such as cutting. A family member or guardian of
the patient should also be interviewed or contacted immediately
if one is not present.

When evaluating a patient who is acutely agitated, attempt
to find out about any precipitating factors, such as a phone
conversation, a visitor, or a conflict with someone on the unit.
This will facilitate supportive interventions that may prevent the
need for medication or restraint. In addition, it will guide you
in alteration of the treatment plan in order to prevent further
episodes.

A consultation on the pediatric floor involves the components
of an evaluation as outlined above. It also includes a review of
the medical chart to assess for medical and metabolic etiologies
of the patient's symptoms.

The interview with any patient should start with nonthreatening questions in order to establish rapport. Begin with questions
about name, age, school, family members, and so forth before
asking about circumstances of the admission. This approach will
be especially helpful with children.

Suicide

When suicide is the chief complaint, it must be taken very
seriously. This is especially true of children and adolescents, who
do not usually choose to visit the hospital but are brought in
by adults for evaluation. Even if the suicide attempt appears
manipulative, it should be regarded as extremely serious. As with
adults, try to ascertain why the attempt was made. Was it related
to a mood disturbance, intoxication, psychosis or command auditory hallucinations, or abuse? This may be easier to determine
with adolescents than with children.

Try to assess the seriousness of the attempt. Was it planned?
Did anyone know? Was anyone present? Where did it happen?
What did the patient take, and how much? If it was an attempt
to jump out a window, what floor was it on? What did the patient
think would happen? Was the patient sick or injured? Could the
patient have died? Did the patient want to die? Is there a gun in
the home, or is one available to the patient?

It is useful to know the child's understanding of death. Ask
the following questions: Is death permanent or reversible? Where
do you go when you die? Do you know anyone who has died or
committed suicide, especially in the family?

If the attempt was impulsive, try to assess whether it might happen again. Is there evidence of other impulsive behaviors?

Aggression/Homicidal Ideation

Try to understand the underlying problem. Is there a specific stressor? Is the behavior directed at one person? Is the aggression apparent in school, at home, or in other spheres? How dangerous is the aggression for the patient or others? Is it the result of a mood disturbance, psychosis, intoxication, or physical and/or sexual abuse? Is it a symptom of organic brain syndrome, mental retardation, autism, or behavioral syndromes? Is the aggression a manifestation of conduct disorder?

Ask about the following:

- Aggression toward people or animals
- Carrying weapons
- Destroying property
- Setting fires
- Deceitfulness or theft
- Serious violations of rules
- Running away from home
- Truancy

To rule out ADHD, ask about difficulties with attention, hyperactivity, and impulsivity both in school and at home.

Psychosis

Psychotic symptoms, such as command auditory hallucinations, can produce unpredictable behavior. Therefore, it is very important to ask about these symptoms in terms that children can understand. Many children do not know the word *hallucination*. They may not understand questions such as "Do you ever see things that are not really there?" A review of systems approach is more useful. For example, ask whether their eyes or ears ever play tricks on them, and give them an example, such as "Do you ever hear someone talking to you when you are in a room all by yourself?" "Do you hear someone talk to you and turn around, but there is nobody there?"

Ask about all of the psychotic symptoms, especially for command auditory hallucinations. Ask the patient when the hallucinations occur, how often they occur, and when they began. Ask if the patient ever feels compelled to act on the command of hallucinations.

■ MANAGEMENT

For emergency room consultations, the physician on call is usually concerned with the evaluation and disposition of the patient rather than with ongoing treatment. What is your formulation? Do you think that the patient requires hospitalization? Discuss the case with a supervisor, an attending physician, or a child and adolescent psychiatry fellow. There are three outcomes to consider: admission, referral, and reports to agencies.

Reports to agencies for neglect and abuse should be discussed with the supervisor and social worker. Different jurisdictions may have somewhat different rules and procedures for this. Also, refer to Appendix L on physical and behavioral indicators of child abuse and neglect to assist you in the evaluation.

If the patient does not require hospitalization but needs follow-up, find an appropriate clinic or referral. If it is too late in the day to make an appointment, tell the parent or legal guardian to be sure to make an appointment the following day. You may wish to take the telephone numbers of the guardian and the referral so that you can arrange for follow-up during the day.

If the patient requires admission, explain to the parent or legal guardian why the patient requires hospitalization. It is important for the parent or legal guardian to understand why the decision was made and that it is in the best interest of the patient. If you take the time to speak with the parents, answer their questions, and listen to their concerns, they are more likely to agree to a voluntary admission. If the patient is likely to become assaultive or try to leave when told of the decision to admit, you may opt to wait until everything is processed and the escort is already present before telling the patient.

You may need to write initial orders for the patient depending on procedures at your hospital. Think about whether the patient will require one-to-one observation in the hospital setting and as-needed (PRN) medication.

Management of acute agitation should be as conservative as possible, while maintaining both the patient's and others' safety. Attempts to calm the patient by supportive verbal intervention should be done first. A mental status examination can help the clinician determine the precipitant for the agitation (e.g., psychosis, suicidal ideation, or acute reaction to a stressor). Separating the patient from the agitating stimulus (e.g., the parent/guardian) is frequently helpful. If available, a quiet room may also be considered for the patient. However, seclusion and restraint policies for children and adolescents should be reviewed for the given institution.

Medications for agitation should only rarely be given to young children. Temper tantrums usually stop before any medication takes effect. A commonly used agent for agitation in both children and adolescents is **diphenhydramine (Benadryl)**, which is approved for use in infants over 20 pounds. Give **25 to 50 mg by mouth (PO) every 2 to 4 hours** until a therapeutic effect is observed, but note that behavioral activation or even hallucinations can sometimes occur, so caution should be used with repeated dosing. Children may require only 25 mg per dose, whereas adolescents may require 50 mg. Diphenhydramine is also available intramuscularly (IM) if needed for severe agitation and can be dosed similarly to oral dosages.

If diphenhydramine is not effective, **lorazepam (Ativan)** can be used. It is approved for children 12 years and older; in younger ages, it is more likely to cause a disinhibiting effect, so its use should be avoided. It is administered at **2 mg PO or 1 to 2 mg IM**. Lorazepam should be avoided in pregnancy.

Haloperidol (Haldol) is approved for children 3 years and older. For acute management of psychotic agitation, use **0.01 to 0.05 mg/kg PO (or half the dosage IM) every 2 to 4 hours** until there is a therapeutic response or side effects are observed.

Chlorpromazine (Thorazine) is approved for use for children 6 months and older. For treatment of psychotic or extremely severe agitation, use **0.25 to 1.0 mg/kg PO every 4 to 6 hours** until there is a therapeutic response or side effects are seen. **Common dosages for adolescents are 25 to 50 mg PO**. If the patient refuses oral medication, **0.5 mg/kg IM** may be administered. Even for a large adolescent, a single IM dose of chlorpromazine should not exceed 50 mg. In children up to 5 years or 50 pounds, the maximum IM daily dose is 40 mg/day; and in children between 5 and 12 years or 50 to 100 pounds, the maximum IM daily dose is 75 mg/day. Be sure to monitor the patient's blood pressure, as hypotension and orthostasis may occur, which puts the patient at risk for falling or even stroke.

When prescribing any of these drugs, remember to check for allergies, previous reactions, medical conditions, and other medications that may be contraindications for their use. Diphenhydramine is likely to have the fewest side effects in medicating an agitated child because there is no risk of dystonia, neuroleptic malignant syndrome, or tardive dyskinesia.

PATIENT-RELATED PROBLEMS: THE COMMON CALLS

8 | The Agitated Patient

Elisabeth Weinstein

Agitation is a clinical state characterized by excessive psycho-motor activity and subjective emotional distress. It can be caused by a myriad of psychiatric and medical illnesses. Motor activity ranges from fidgeting, restlessness, and pacing to threatening and aggressive behavior, which can put both the patient and staff in danger. Motor activities may be accompanied by psychic phenomena, including excitement, confusion, fear, anger, or paranoia. It is very common to be called to evaluate an agitated patient on a medical, surgical, or psychiatric ward.

Your primary goal upon arriving is to assess for potential dangerous behavior and to ensure the safety of the environment for everyone. Secondarily, your goal is to evaluate the patient in order to diagnose and treat the underlying cause of the agitation.

■ PHONE CALL

Questions

1. **What is the nature and duration of the agitation?**
   - What behavior has the patient exhibited?
   - Has the patient displayed similar behavior in the recent past?
   - How was it managed?
   - Is the patient a threat to self, staff, or other patients?
   - Is the patient jeopardizing his or her medical care?
2. **What is the patient's medical history?**
   - What are the vital signs?
   - Does the patient have medical problems?
   - Has there been a change in the level of consciousness?
   - What medications is the patient on? Was any new medication recently started?
3. **What is the patient's psychiatric history?**
   - What is the admission diagnosis?
   - Does the patient have a history of substance abuse?

Orders

1. Order appropriate observation and measurement of vital signs.

2. For an alert, cooperative patient, consider ordering oral medication as needed (PRN) to help with symptomatic relief until you can evaluate the patient. Order low doses so that the patient will be alert for an evaluation when you arrive at the site.
3. If there is an acute danger to the patient or staff members, you will need to order physical or chemical restraints over the telephone. If this is the case, a psychiatric code should be called to alert additional staff that help is needed.

Inform RN

"Will arrive in . . . minutes."

■ ELEVATOR THOUGHTS

What causes agitation?

- The timing of the onset of the agitation provides important information regarding the underlying etiology. A more acute onset may suggest a medical problem. Manic symptoms usually escalate over time, and schizophrenic decompensation usually follows a prodromal period. Substance withdrawal syndromes usually occur 1 to 7 days after admission and are generally accompanied by changes in vital signs.
- An assessment of the level of consciousness may also help elucidate the underlying cause of an agitated state. Patients who are agitated because of a primary psychiatric illness should have no fluctuation in level of consciousness and should be fully alert. Patients who are agitated because of a primary medical illness frequently will have fluctuations in their level of consciousness and may not be alert.
- A good history and physical examination will help elucidate the underlying cause of an agitated state. Someone with multiple medical problems or taking multiple medications is more likely to have a general medical condition causing the agitation. Likewise, someone who appears to be in physical distress usually has a medical condition causing the agitation. Be sure to assess fall risk and rule out recent head injury as a cause of symptoms.

Psychiatric Causes of Agitation

- Psychotic disorders
- Mood disorders
- Anxiety disorders
- Personality disorders

Medical Causes of Agitation

1. **Systemic**
   a. **Metabolic**
      (1) Electrolyte imbalances
      (2) Diabetes
      (3) Hypoxia
      (4) Acute intermittent porphyria
   b. **Endocrine**
      (1) Thyroid and adrenal conditions
      (2) Carcinoid syndrome
   c. **Organ failure**
      (1) Hepatic encephalopathy
      (2) Uremic encephalopathy
      (3) Respiratory failure
      (4) Cardiovascular conditions
         (a) Congestive heart failure
         (b) Coronary artery disease
         (c) Paroxysmal supraventricular tachycardia and other arrhythmias

2. **Drugs**
   a. **Drugs of abuse**
      (1) Alcohol intoxication, delirium, and withdrawal (one of the most common causes of postoperative agitation is alcohol withdrawal)
      (2) Stimulant intoxication and withdrawal
      (3) Sedative, hypnotic, and anxiolytic withdrawal and delirium
   b. **Idiosyncratic or toxic effects of medications**
      (1) Corticosteroids
      (2) Anticholinergic medications
      (3) Anticonvulsants
      (4) Antihistamines
      (5) Antimalarials
      (6) Antibiotics
      (7) Others: lidocaine, meperidine, metoclopramide, podophyllin, procaine penicillin, propoxiphene withdrawal, pyridostigmine, and sulfonamides
   c. **Idiosyncratic or side effects of psychotropics**
      (1) Benzodiazepine withdrawal or disinhibition (especially in patients with organic disease)
      (2) L-dopa
      (3) Antidepressants: tricyclic, selective, and nonselective serotonin reuptake inhibitors and monoamine oxidase inhibitors
      (4) Antipsychotics: akathisia?
      (5) Psychostimulants

d. **Poisonings**
   (1) Carbon monoxide
   (2) Insecticides
3. **Central nervous system**
   a. **Trauma**
      (1) Subdural and epidural hematoma
      (2) Hemorrhage
   b. **Vascular conditions**
      (1) Transient ischemic attack
      (2) Stroke
      (3) Vasculitis: systemic lupus erythematosus and polyarteritis nodosa
   c. **Infections**
      (1) Meningitis
      (2) Encephalitis
      (3) Human immunodeficiency virus (HIV) and aquired immunodeficiency syndrome (AIDS)–related conditions
      (4) Lyme disease
   d. **Epilepsy**
      (1) Complex partial seizure disorder
      (2) Postictal states
   e. **Dementia:** age and diagnosis are important ("sundowning" is a common cause of agitation in older patients but is a diagnosis of exclusion)
      (1) Alzheimer's disease
      (2) Multi-infarct dementia: hypertension, stepwise progression, and focal necrologic signs
      (3) Normal-pressure hydrocephalus: dementia, gait apraxia, and incontinence
      (4) Parkinson's disease
      (5) Other: Vitamin B_{12} deficiency, Wernicke-Korsakoff syndrome, Huntington's disease, Pick's disease, and multiple sclerosis
      (6) Neoplasms
      (7) Hypertensive encephalopathy

■ MAJOR THREAT TO LIFE

- The most common immediate risk with an agitated patient is the potential for aggression from lack of behavioral control. Agitated patients can have tremendous strength and can hit or throw things, making it dangerous to be in their presence.
- Agitation can also be physically uncomfortable for the patient. Akathisia, for example, can even increase the risk of suicide.
- Agitation may be the first sign of a potentially life-threatening

medical condition (e.g., intracranial bleeding or tumor, pulmonary embolism, myocardial infarct, hypoglycemia, neuroleptic malignant syndrome).

- Untreated agitation can lead to serious medical complications, including exhaustion, dehydration, rhabdomyolysis, renal failure, and even death.

■ BEDSIDE

Depending on the degree and nature of the agitation, there may or may not be time to go through the medical chart. The patient should be evaluated first to assess whether there is time to review the patient's medical records.

Quick Look Test

The patient should be initially viewed from a distance. If the patient appears to be in control and able to cooperate, you can approach him or her cautiously in order to perform an evaluation. If the patient appears to be in distress or has a significant amount of psychomotor activity, you should assume that the situation may be dangerous and prepare for it before approaching the patient.

Some guidelines include the following:
1. Make sure there is a sufficient number of trained staff members available to help physically control the patient. A show of force may help prevent aggressive behaviors.
2. Do not wear loose hair, hanging clothing (ties), or exposed jewelry that a patient can grab.
3. Assess the environment for dangerous objects and remove them.
4. Do not place yourself in a situation or room where the patient can trap or assault you. Stand closer to the door than the patient stands or evaluate the patient in an open space.
5. Separate the agitated patient from an overstimulating situation.
6. Avoid getting too close to the patient.
7. Use clear and direct language to avoid ambiguity.
8. When approaching the agitated patient, avoid threatening behavior and remain calm in voice and demeanor.

■ MANAGEMENT
Initial Management

1. If the patient is able to cooperate with an interview, he or she can be evaluated in a quiet, open area that is easily accessible

to nursing staff. Sometimes an agitated patient can get relief by explaining what he or she is experiencing or from a calming, supportive interaction. Time in a quiet room can be suggested, and this too can be helpful. Frequently oral medication PRN can be helpful in relieving agitation in a nonacute situation. These measures are particularly useful for patients with personality and anxiety disorders. They tend to be less helpful for acutely psychotic, manic, or medically ill patients.

2. If the patient is out of control or unable to respond to the above measures, the situation can become quickly dangerous, and physical or chemical restraint may be necessary to keep the patient and the environment safe. This is common with acutely manic or psychotic patients.

3. If the patient is experiencing obvious physical symptoms (e.g., cyanosis, shortness of breath, pain, sweating, tremulousness), acknowledgment of the problem and immediate intervention will reduce the patient's level of agitation. Obtaining vital signs is absolutely necessary with the physically compromised patient. A hypoxic patient should respond to oxygen, and a hypoglycemic patient should respond to glucose. If the patient's condition is unimproved by your interventions, call for medical backup.

4. Patients on medical and surgical wards often exhibit agitated behavior, which can compromise their medical care. Once this is evident, restraint is indicated. Hesitation may jeopardize the patient's safety and care.

5. The following is a general strategy for the initial management of an agitated patient:
   a. Attempt to verbally redirect the patient by talking him or her down and setting firm limits.
   b. Offer oral medication.
   c. If the patient resists your efforts and continues to be agitated, consider seclusion, restraint, and/or intramuscular medications.

Continued Management

1. After emergency measures are carried out, read the chart and follow up with the staff and the patient to determine further treatment. This should include gathering a complete psychiatric and medical history. Any interventions should reinforce the existing treatment plan.

2. A physical examination should be performed, with attention to neurologic assessment.

3. Laboratory tests should be ordered and followed up to facilitate treatment of underlying medical conditions. Consider obtaining the following:

a. Complete blood count
b. Electrolytes
c. Liver function tests
d. Thyroid function tests
e. Serum alcohol and urine toxicologies
f. Arterial blood gas
g. Medication levels (if suspect, hold medication until further notice)
h. Electrocardiogram (ECG)
i. Electroencephalogram (EEG)
j. Skull or head imaging
4. Do not hesitate to call other consultants if you suspect medical conditions.
5. If the agitation is thought to be due to medication toxicity, consider discontinuing, tapering, or adding medications. Stopping or decreasing doses of medications may not immediately relieve the agitation, and therefore psychotropics may initially be required to control the agitation. In some cases, more aggressive interventions may be indicated (e.g., toxic lithium levels may require intravenous [IV] fluids or even renal dialysis). Sudden discontinuation of certain medications may have deleterious effects. To ensure good follow-up, document your consultation and the rationale for your decisions.
6. In cases of suspected overdose, follow protocols for the specific substance.

■ MEDICATING THE PATIENT

Generally, you may prescribe haloperidol for the psychotic agitated patient and lorazepam for the nonpsychotic agitated patient. Both of these medications can be given intramuscularly (IM) if needed. Small doses of atypical antipsychotics are frequently given to the agitated geriatric patient as they are often better tolerated. Small doses of an antipsychotic can be given in conjunction with benzodiazepines to prevent disinhibition in patients with this tendency. This combination can also prevent dystonias caused by antipsychotics. The following are usual doses (doses should be adjusted for geriatric and medically compromised patients):

1. **Haloperidol 5 mg orally (PO) or IM can be given every 30 minutes** until the patient is calmed down. Contraindications include a history of neuroleptic malignant syndrome or laryngeal dystonias. Remember that antipsychotics can lower the seizure threshold.
2. **Benztropine 2 mg IM** can be initially administered with haloperidol to prevent side effects. **Diphenhydramine 25 to 50 mg IM** can also be used. Benztropine or diphenhydra-

mine can be repeated in 10 minutes or less if side effects are still distressful or life threatening.

3. **Lorazepam 2 mg PO or IM can be repeated every 30 minutes** and can be used in conjunction with haloperidol.

The following are alternative medications:

1. **Chlorpromazine 100 to 200 mg PO or 25 to 50 mg IM** can be administered. Extreme caution should be used with IM chlorpromazine because of the potential for orthostatic hypotension and therefore do not give IM injections over 50 mg.

2. **Diphenhydramine 50 mg PO or IM** can be given to patients sensitive to antipsychotics or benzodiazepines. It can also be used to control agitation in children.

3. **Amytal Sodium 50 to 250 mg PO or IM** has limited applications and can cause severe orthostasis. This drug is contraindicated for patients with acute intermittent porphyria.

It is best to stay on the ward until the agitation has been resolved in order to observe the mental status of the patient and to support the staff.

9 | The Anxious Patient

PATRICK YING

Anxiety is characterized by a feeling of fear accompanied by physical signs indicative of a hyperactive autonomic nervous system. When evaluating the anxious patient, the clinician must distinguish between normal and pathologic anxiety states. Normal anxiety is a universal, possibly advantageous response to threats, challenges, or uncertainty. In contrast, pathologic anxiety, with respect to its intensity, duration, or character, is an inappropriate response given a particular stimulus; in fact, often no external stimulus can be identified. The clinician must also distinguish primary anxiety from anxiety secondary to medical disease or substance/medication use. Anxiety of sufficient intensity to necessitate an emergency room visit or a call from staff nurses will require a careful medical and psychiatric evaluation with appropriate treatment. It may be tempting to attribute the symptoms of anxiety to a known psychiatric disorder. It is imperative, however, that the clinician rule out underlying medical problems or substance/medication use.

■ PHONE CALL

Questions

1. What are the patient's presenting symptoms?
2. Does the patient have any medical illnesses?
3. What medications is the patient taking?
4. Does the patient have a history of drug or alcohol abuse?
5. Does the patient have a history of a psychiatric disorder?
6. What are the vital signs?

Orders

1. The most important aspect of assessment over the telephone is to recognize if the patient is in a life-threatening situation. You should have some idea about the nature of the patient's symptoms from the nurses' responses to your initial questions. Order the vital signs if they were not already taken.

2. Although it is not usual practice to order medications over the telephone, this may be indicated in certain situations. For example, a wheezing patient with a known history of asthma may benefit from as-needed (PRN) medications for asthma before your arrival.
3. Place the patient in a safe and quiet environment.
4. As fear is a major component of anxiety, make sure that the patient is being closely observed and attended to.
5. Based on the patient's symptoms, ask the nursing staff to have an electrocardiograph available or to perform an electrocardiogram (ECG) before you arrive.

Inform RN

"Will arrive in . . . minutes."

After the telephone call, prioritize your arrival depending on the severity of the patient's symptoms. If the cardiovascular or respiratory system is the suspected etiology, see the patient immediately. If the patient's vital signs are stable and the situation is not life threatening, your arrival is less urgent.

■ ELEVATOR THOUGHTS

What causes anxiety?
- Physical problems (Table 9–1)
- Drug-related problems (Table 9–2)
- Primary psychiatric disorders
  Generalized anxiety disorder (GAD)
  Panic disorder
  Phobia
  Obsessive-compulsive disorder (OCD)
  Post-traumatic stress disorder (PTSD)
  Adjustment disorder with anxiety
  Cluster B or C personality disorder
- Akathisia
- Anxiety secondary to psychotic symptoms
- Anxiety in the context of depressive disorders

■ MAJOR THREAT TO LIFE

Untreated anxiety can be disabling and can lead to impaired judgment. When anxiety becomes intolerable, as can happen in panic disorder, PTSD, and akathisia, it has been associated with suicidal behavior. When substance abuse complicates anxiety, overdoses are common. In addition, anxiety can be a symptom of alcohol withdrawal, which can lead to delirium tremens if not

Table 9–1 □ PHYSICAL CAUSES OF ANXIETY-LIKE SYMPTOMS

Type of Cause	Specific Cause
Cardiovascular	Angina pectoris, arrhythmias, congestive heart failure, hypertension, hypovolemia, myocardial infarction, syncope (multiple causes), valvular disease, vascular collapse (shock)
Dietary	Caffeine, monosodium glutamate (Chinese restaurant syndrome), vitamin-deficiency diseases
Drug related	Akathisia (secondary to antipsychotic drugs), anticholinergic toxicity, digitalis toxicity, hallucinogens, hypotensive agents, stimulants (amphetamines, cocaine, related drugs), withdrawal syndromes (alcohol, sedative-hypnotics), bronchodilators (theophylline, sympathomimetics)
Hematologic	Anemias
Immunologic	Anaphylaxis, systemic lupus erythematosus
Metabolic	Hyperadrenalism (Cushing's disease), hyperkalemia, hyperthermia, hyperthyroidism, hypocalcemia, hypoglycemia, hyponatremia, hypothyroidism, menopause, porphyria (acute intermittent)
Neurologic	Encephalopathies (infectious, metabolic, toxic), essential tremor, intracranial mass lesions, postconcussive syndrome, seizure disorders (especially of the temporal lobe), vertigo
Respiratory	Asthma, chronic obstructive pulmonary disease, pneumonia, pneumothorax, pulmonary edema, pulmonary embolism
Secreting tumors	Carcinoid, insulinoma, pheochromocytoma

From Rosenbaum JF: The drug treatment of anxiety. N Engl J Med 1982; 306:401. Copyright 1982 Massachusetts Medical Society. All rights reserved.

treated appropriately. It is imperative for you to consider the medical causes of anxiety because they may result in significant morbidity or mortality if left untreated.

■ BEDSIDE

Quick Look Test

What are the patient's facial expression, posture, and mannerisms?

These may give indications of the patient's level of anxiety.

Table 9–2 □ DRUGS THAT MAY CAUSE ANXIETY

Stimulants	**Anticholinergics**
Amphetamine	Benztropine mesylate (Cogentin)
Aminophylline	Diphenhydramine (Benadryl)
Caffeine	Meperidine (Demerol)
Cocaine	Oxybutynin (Ditropan)
Methylphenidate	Propantheline (Probanthine)
Theophylline	Tricyclics
	Trihexyphenidyl (Artane)
Sympathomimetics	
Ephedrine	**Dopaminergics**
Epinephrine	Amantadine
Phenylpropanolamine	Antipsychotics
Pseudoephedrine	Bromocriptine
	Levodopa (L-dopa)
Drug Withdrawal	Levodopa-carbidopa (Sinemet)
Barbiturates	Metoclopramide
Benzodiazepines	
Narcotics	**Miscellaneous**
Alcohol	Baclofen
Sedative	Cycloserine
	Hallucinogens
	Indomethacin

From Goldberg RJ: Practical Guide to the Care of the Psychiatric Patient. St. Louis, Mosby–Year Book, 1995.

Is the patient breathing in a fast and shallow manner, clutching his or her throat? Is the patient holding his or her chest or abdomen, sweating, or holding on to an object, fearing that he or she might collapse?

These patients are generally receptive to any support that you have to offer and even in the middle of an attack will be able to verbalize their symptoms.

Is the patient describing dizziness, faintness, fear of going crazy, or even fear of dying?

Be sure to carefully examine the patient because these symptoms can mimic medical problems.

Is the patient pacing? Is the patient fidgety and unable to sit or stand still?

These signs can also indicate that a patient is experiencing akathisia.

On occasion, you may arrive to find the patient calm, relaxed, and able to describe symptoms in a coherent manner because acute anxiety attacks can be self-limited. Do not be misled by rapid relief from symptoms and withhold treatment or a careful examination.

Airway and Vital Signs

Although the RN should have already taken vital signs, it is advisable to order vital signs to be taken frequently. This may have a calming effect on the patient as well.

Selective History and Chart Review

The onset of the anxiety and the precipitating and alleviating factors help to determine the cause as either a primary psychiatric disturbance or a condition secondary to a medical condition or drug. A patient with no prior history of anxiety merits a full psychiatric and medical evaluation. Do not ascribe anxiety to a medical problem unless the available data, signs, and symptoms point to a medical etiology. In this case, perform the relevant physical examination and indicated laboratory work to rule out suspected medical problems. The medical history is very important, as is the list of medications and dosages. Common issues to consider are the following:

1. Whether the patient is overusing medications that can produce anxiety, such as bronchodilators
2. Whether the patient is experiencing side effects of drug interactions, such as with fluoxetine or cimetidine, which inhibit the cytochrome P450 system and may increase the plasma levels of other drugs such as digoxin
3. Whether there have been recent changes in medication, either additions or subtractions, that might be responsible for the onset of anxiety

When patients begin new medications, anxiety may be a direct side effect or simply a reaction to having to take a new medication. In particular with patients taking antipsychotics (and, to a lesser degree, selective serotonin reuptake inhibitors [SSRIs]), the possibility of akathisia must be entertained. Akathisia is characterized by a subjective feeling of restlessness, especially in the lower extremities, and an inability to sit or stand still. Although akathisia is more likely to occur soon after initiation or increase of the medication, it can occur at any time during treatment. Akathisia is frequently misdiagnosed as anxiety or agitation; it may be distinguished from anxiety as being a restlessness that stems from the muscles instead of from the mind, and patients may feel worse if asked to sit or stand still. Recognition of akathisia is important, as misdiagnosis could lead to increasing the dosage of the antipsychotic (or SSRI), which would make the symptoms worse.

Abrupt discontinuation of medications such as benzodiazepines or antidepressants can provoke withdrawal that can cause anxiety. In particular, antidepressants with shorter half-lives such as venlafaxine, fluvoxamine and paroxetine are more prone to discontinuation syndromes, which can include dizziness, lethargy, headache, irritability, and anxiety.

When evaluating an anxious patient, it is important that you obtain a drug and alcohol history, including caffeine-containing and over-the-counter products (e.g., cold remedies). Dietary supplements for weight loss or weight gain, herbal medications, and other alternative or "natural" products often contain stimulants and sympathomimetics, such as ephedrine (look for ingredients called ephedra or ma-huang), and can precipitate anxiety, especially in high doses. If substance abuse is suspected, order a urine toxicology screen and treat accordingly. Some patients who abuse substances exaggerate symptoms in order to gain access to more drugs. It is also common, however, that patients who abuse substances are self-medicating an underlying anxiety disorder. It can be helpful in these cases to look for objective signs of anxiety and to discuss with the staff if the patient's behavior before your arrival has been consistent with anxiety.

Mental Status Examination

Although the full mental status examination is important, some features are more relevant to anxiety. An anxious patient's appearance, posture, gestures, and facial expressions are revealing. Motor behavior may reveal agitation and restlessness. Also note any sweating or tremulousness (speech may be stammering or stuttering). Mood and affect usually reflect anxiety. Thought processes may still remain logical. Although there are usually no perceptual disturbances, the use of substances may induce them. Psychotic symptoms can certainly provoke anxiety. There may be depersonalization and derealization. Sensorium is generally clear. Cognition may appear impaired secondary to the level of distress. For the same reason, the patient's insight and judgment may also appear impaired.

Selective Physical Examination

The physical examination can be helpful in identifying a medical etiology for anxiety. First, the physical examination should be directed toward evaluating somatic complaints that the patient offers and any pre-existing medical conditions that could contribute to anxiety in order to rule out a possible medical etiology. A neurologic examination, including examination of the pupils, deep tendon reflexes, and tremors, can pick up signs of substance abuse or withdrawal. Patients with akathisia can have characteristic objective signs such as swinging of one leg while sitting, or rocking from foot to foot or "walking on the spot" while standing.

■ MANAGEMENT

The most important aspect of the management of the anxious patient is to address contributing medical problems, if any. Providing a secure and safe environment for the patient is also important and often includes ensuring a quiet and nonstimulating area, with intermittent observation. You and the nursing staff should allow the anxious patient to express his or her concerns. This intervention alone may alleviate the patient's anxiety.

The next step is to check that there are no medications responsible for inducing the anxiety, as well as no history of substance abuse. In the case of substance-induced or medication-induced anxiety, withholding the offending agent should alleviate the symptoms. In the case of akathisia, if possible, lower the dose of the antipsychotic medication. Next, consider a beta-blocker. Typically, **propranolol (Inderal), starting at 10 mg orally (PO) three times a day,** is used. If beta-blockers are contraindicated, second-line treatments include anticholinergics such as **benztropine (Cogentin) 0.5 to 1 mg PO or intramuscularly (IM) every 6 hours** and **clonidine (Catapress) 0.05 to 0.1 mg PO every 12 hours** may be used instead. Benzodiazepines are also useful as a second-line treatment or as an adjunctive treatment especially if the patient is in great distress. Anxiety induced by either substance abuse or withdrawal should be approached as medically indicated.

In other cases of anxiety, the next step should be to assess the need for medication. Reassuring the patient, identifying the cause of the anxiety, and teaching basic relaxation techniques such as deep diaphragmatic breathing may be adequate interventions. Even if nonpharmacologic interventions have been somewhat effective, however, the patient may still benefit from medication, especially when the anxiety is likely to persist or to interfere with other care the patient is receiving. In general, the benzodiazepines are the most effective drugs for the treatment of acute anxiety. The patient who is anxious secondary to psychotic symptoms may also benefit from additional neuroleptic medication, such as a PRN dose of **haloperidol 0.5 to 5 mg PO/IM**. Before you initiate any pharmacologic strategy, consider drug interactions, side effects, and contraindications. Important points to keep in mind when administering benzodiazepines include the following:

1. Behavioral disinhibition can occur.
2. Possible respiratory depression can occur in compromised individuals.
3. Addiction and withdrawal syndromes can occur.
4. Hepatic dysfunction and some medications can inhibit the metabolism (oxidation) of certain benzodiazepines. Lorazepam, tempazepam, and oxazepam are least affected by these interactions.

Table 9-3 □ DATA ON AVAILABLE BENZODIAZEPINES

Available Preparations	Oral Dosage Equivalency (mg)	Onset After Oral Dose	Distribution Half-life	Elimination Half-life (hr)*
Alprazolam [Xanax]	0.5	Intermediate	Intermediate	6–20
Chlordiazepoxide [Librium and generics]	10.0	Intermediate	Slow	30–100
Clonazepam [Klonopin]	0.25	Intermediate	Intermediate	18–50
Clorazepate [Tranxene]†	7.5	Rapid	Rapid	30–100
Diazepam [Valium and generics]	5.0	Rapid	Rapid	30–100
Estazolam [ProSom]	2.0	Intermediate	Intermediate	10–24
Flurazepam [Dalmane]	30.0	Rapid to intermediate	Rapid	50–160
Lorazepam [Ativan and generics]	1.0	Intermediate	Intermediate	10–20
Midazolam [Versed]	—	Intermediate	Rapid	2–3
Oxazepam [Serax]	15.0	Intermediate to slow	Intermediate	8–12
Quazepam [Doral]	15.0	Rapid to intermediate	Intermediate	50–160
Temazepam [Restoril]	30.0	Intermediate	Rapid	8–20
Triazolam [Halcion]	0.25	Intermediate	Rapid	1.5–5

*The elimination half-life represents the total for all active metabolites; the elderly tend to have the longer half-lives in the ranges reported. Chlordiazepoxide, clorazepate, and diazepam have desmethyldiazepam as a long-lived active metabolite. Flurazepam and quazepam share N-desalkylflurazepam as a long-lived active metabolite. With chronic dosing, these active metabolites represent most of the pharmacodynamic effect of these drugs
†Clorazepate is an inactive prodrug for desmethyldiazepam, which is the active compound in the blood.
From Hyman S, Arana GW, Rosenbaum JF (eds): Handbook of Psychiatric Drug Therapy, 3rd Edition. Boston, Little, Brown, and Company, 1995.

5. Benzodiazepines act synergistically with other central nervous system depressants (narcotics, barbiturates, alcohol).
6. Side effects can occur, including cognitive impairment, confusion, disorientation, psychomotor impairment, drowsiness, and depressive symptoms, especially in the elderly.

If the patient has a history of a good response to a specific benzodiazepine, instituting the same medication is usually the best idea (Table 9–3). There are many benzodiazepines available, but lorazepam (Ativan) is often the drug of choice to medicate acute anxiety. Lorazepam, unlike some other benzodiazepines, is well absorbed and easily administered IM or IV. Such parenteral routes are often needed in acute situations. Lorazepam also has a fairly rapid onset of action and is less affected by hepatic difficulties and drug interactions than are many other benzodiazepines. **Lorazepam can be given in doses of 1 to 2 mg PO/IM/IV and may be repeated every 30 minutes several times** if clinical response has not been achieved.

If the patient's anxiety does not respond after multiple doses, one must reconsider the diagnosis and treatment. At this point, possible medical etiologies should again be reviewed, especially substance abuse or withdrawal, akathisia, and medical problems. As well, patients with a history of benzodiazepine treatment may have a degree of tolerance and therefore require higher doses for effect. If the patient shows signs of paradoxical disinhibition, additional benzodiazepines should not be given. Second-line pharmacologic therapies should be considered, including antihistamines, such as hydroxyzine and diphenhydramine, beta-blockers, and low-dose antipsychotics, especially if behavioral dyscontrol is marked.

10 | The Violent Patient

MICHELLE E. MONTEMAYOR

Often the psychiatric physician receives a request to manage a threatening or dangerous situation already in progress. The patient may be injuring himself or herself and/or others or may damage property, creating dangerous conditions.

In this chapter, risk assessment and management of the actively dangerous patient are discussed. The identification and management of potentially violent patients are also covered.

■ PHONE CALL

Questions

The context in which you are called to evaluate the patient is important in making the assessment of dangerousness. Is this an initial emergency room evaluation, or is the patient admitted on a hospital ward?

1. **What is the acuity of the situation?**
   - Is the patient verbally threatening?
   - Has the situation escalated to physical assaultiveness?
   - Is the violent behavior toward self or other?
   - Have other patients or staff been injured?
   - Does the patient have a weapon?
   - Does the patient have a history of threatening behavior or physical attacks?
2. **What is the reason for presentation to the emergency room?**
   - Is the patient intoxicated or withdrawing from illicit drugs or alcohol?
   - Has the patient engaged in assaultive behavior immediately before this incident (i.e., in police custody for assault)?
3. **Is the patient able to respond to verbal redirection?**
   - Has oral medication been offered?
   - Has the patient been moved to an area with minimal environmental stimulation?
   - Has one-to-one staff supervision been instituted?
4. **If the patient is unable or unwilling to respond verbally, has hospital security been called to assist in bringing**

the patient under control for administration of intramuscular medication and/or seclusion and restraints?
5. Once the violent situation has been managed appropriately, how would you characterize the cause(s) and
duration of the threatening behavior?
   - What is the source of the patient's distress?
   - Is the patient expressing ongoing violent behavior, or is
     this an isolated incident?

Orders

1. When the patient acts in a manner that jeopardizes the safety
   of self and/or others, call hospital security to subdue the
   patient. In most cases, a show of force (i.e., arrival of several
   members of the security team at one time) is enough to
   persuade the patient to respond to verbal redirection before
   your arrival.
2. Ask the nurse to make restraints and PRN intramuscular
   medication available. If the level of dangerousness is
   deemed significant, give verbal orders to execute these measures as soon as adequate staff support arrives. Ideally, you
   will be present to evaluate and direct these measures as they
   are instituted.

Inform RN

"Will arrive in . . . minutes."
Threatening and/or violent behavior necessitates a decisive
and immediate response.

■ ELEVATOR THOUGHTS

As the psychiatric physician called to assess a dangerous situation, your attitude can facilitate the neutralization of a violent
incident. Recognition of the emotionally charged circumstances
you are about to face is often helpful to set the tone for this
difficult interaction. Remain as calm as possible, and speak slowly
and softly, but firmly and clearly. Be as respectful as possible to
all parties involved.

Causes of violent behavior are complex and multidimensional;
demographics, psychiatric and medical factors, family history,
social history, history of assault, and the particular situation at
hand may all play a role in the current situation. The single best
predictor of future violence is past violence. If a patient has an
established history of violent behavior, proceed with caution.

With respect to demographics, the violent patient is more likely
to be a young male, roughly 18 to 25 years old, having a low

socioeconomic status and limited social supports. Race has not been found to correlate with violence when socioeconomic status is controlled for.

Axis I psychiatric diagnoses are correlated with higher incidences of violent behavior. In particular, patients with a history of violent behavior have been diagnosed with schizophrenia, schizoaffective disorder, major depressive disorder, bipolar disorder, obsessive-compulsive disorder, and panic disorder. Substance dependence or abuse is associated with a likelihood of past violent behavior to a greater extent than other Axis I diagnoses are. For patients with a dual diagnosis, the history of violence is compounded to an even higher percentage of the population. Recognition and treatment of underlying psychiatric or medical causes of threatening assaultive behavior can often ameliorate or eliminate it.

Psychiatric factors that underlie violent behavior include the following:

- Command auditory hallucinations
- Paranoid delusions
- Psychomotor agitation or restlessness
- Hyperarousal or suspiciousness
- Explosive anger or impulsivity
- Disorientation, delirium, or dementia
- Limited mental capacity or mental retardation
- Alcohol and/or illicit substance intoxication or withdrawal
- Psychiatric medication side effect(s) or overdose

Many medical conditions can contribute to violent behavior, including the following:

- Seizure disorder
- History of brain trauma
- Systemic infection
- Hazardous exposure (heavy metals, organic solvents or pesticides)
- Infarct or hemorrhage
- Electrolyte abnormalities
- Vitamin deficiency (B_{12}, thiamine)
- Endocrine disorders
- Hepatic or renal impairment or failure
- Immunologic disorders

■ MAJOR THREAT TO LIFE

- Unrecognized medical or psychiatric problem

  Withdrawal from substances of abuse or other psychiatric or medical conditions may first come to attention in the context of the "violent patient." Although management of the dangerousness is the first priority, be sure to evaluate the patient for signs and symptoms of possible untreated or undertreated medical or psychiatric illness.

- Physical injury

    If a patient is threatening or engaging in harm to self or others, institute one-to-one staff observation of the patient. Take necessary measures to ensure safety. Medication, seclusion, and/or restraint may be involved. It is important to instruct the patient on the level of behavioral control that must be exhibited before discontinuation of orders instituted for the patient's safety. This subject is further elaborated in the chapter on seclusion and restraints.

■ BEDSIDE

Quick Look Test

Always have additional staff present during evaluation of a violent patient. If warranted, wait for the arrival of additional personnel in order to facilitate patient cooperation.

What is the emotional tone of the area?
Is the patient quiet and calm or loud and agitated? How is the staff responding? Has anyone been injured? Does property destruction pose a risk (broken glass, exposed electrical wiring)?

Is the area secure?
Is the patient in possession of a weapon or an object that can be used as one? Have all potential weapons been cleared from the area (light furniture and/or any object that can be picked up and thrown)? Have other patients and those not directly involved with patient care been cleared from the area? Are exits secured (especially important in open emergency room settings)?

What is the patient's mental state?
Does the patient respond to you appropriately (in a related fashion)? Does he or she appear alert and oriented? Is he or she organized in appearance? Is his or her speech pressured, slurred, loud, threatening? Is he or she physically agitated, restless, or pacing? Is he or she tense (hands in fists)?

Are the patient's thought processes appropriate?
Is he or she goal oriented or disorganized? Does he or she appear to be responding to internal stimuli? Is he or she fearful or paranoid? Is some other delusional process evident?

■ MANAGEMENT

Before approaching the patient, remove any neckwear (necktie, scarf, dangling chain, or stethoscope), pens, or other objects you are wearing that can potentially be used as a weapon. Women should not wear dangling pierced earrings that may be torn from the ears. If you choose to wear your hospital identification around your neck, use a break-away chain (these are often provided by hospital security).

Approach the patient slowly, in a relaxed manner, with hands visible. Do not make quick or unexpected movements. Announce your intentions in advance of any action. Always remain at least 3 to 6 feet away from the patient. Stand sideways firmly on your feet so that you can pivot away from a potentially combative patient. This stance offers less of a surface area for attack than a full frontal stance. Do not turn your back on the patient until you are 15 to 20 feet away.

Assess the patient for the possibility that he or she is in possession of a weapon. In the emergency room, patients are usually searched before evaluation. Do not assume that this has been done. Even on the hospital floor, weapon possession is a possibility. If you suspect that the patient has a weapon, ask him or her directly. If you are not satisfied with the response, verbally appeal to the patient to surrender the weapon by placing it on the floor or the desk. Then ask the patient to step away from it. Never ask the patient to hand you a weapon. Never attempt to take a weapon from the patient. When necessary, call hospital security to perform a search.

If the patient is amenable to verbal redirection, invite the patient to sit down with you in an open area and discuss the problem. Check your voice and posture. No matter how agitated the patient is, speak slowly, calmly, and firmly. Make sure that the environment has the least stimuli possible. Give the patient space; you and other staff members should be positioned nearest to the exits.

Often the "violent" patient is fearful or frustrated by his or her situation. He or she may feel abandoned, ridiculed, or misunderstood, and his or her behavior may be a crude attempt to be heard. One of the most effective interventions in such instances is to actively listen to the patient's concerns in a nonjudgmental manner. Ask the patient to describe the trouble. If the patient presents a reasonable request or concern, do what you can to comply or support his or her position. If the patient's wishes are unreasonable or unrealistic, firmly and clearly state the rules. If possible, offer a more reasonable or realistic alternative. Be verbally appreciative of any cooperation you may receive from the staff and the patient.

Even if agitation is present, most patients will comply with your request to discuss the situation. This outcome is much more likely if staff is present in significant number. Encourage the patient to take oral medication to help regain self-control. **Lorazepam (Ativan),** a medium half-life (8 to 20 hours) benzodiazepine, **may be given to the mildly agitated patient in a dose of 1 to 2 mg.** Offering the patient something to eat (a sandwich) helps to restore a calm, receptive mood in many cases. Do not give the patient food items that may be hurled at you.

For the more agitated patient, the sedative effect of a high-potency antipsychotic such as **haloperidol (Haldol) 5 mg** is helpful. It may be added to the benzodiazepine. Avoid extrapyramidal side effects and/or dystonia (especially in the neuroleptic naïve patient) by adding **benztropine mesylate (Cogentin) 1 to 2 mg** or **diphenhydramine (Benadryl) 25 to 50 mg.** When possible, use oral suspensions rather than pills or tablets for better absorption and to minimize the risk of the patient's "cheeking" the medication.

The dose of benzodiazepine or antipsychotic is substantially reduced for elderly, adolescent, live-compromised, and Asian populations. For children, diphenhydramine 25 mg is used as the sole agent to ameliorate agitation. As a rule, when in doubt, start low and go slow.

For the more agitated patient or one who refuses pharmacologic intervention, intramuscular medication may be required. The medications discussed above may be given intramuscularly in similar doses. The degree of agitation or the size of the patient may not be a reliable indicator of the amount of medication that may be needed.

If the patient is combative or threatening violence to self or others, a limited period of restraint may be necessary. Be sure to review the hospital policies and state laws concerning this type of treatment. Document the time started, duration, termination time, and indication for any restraint or seclusion order. Instruct the patient on the necessary verbalization and behavioral control required to terminate these restrictive measures. Document that this instruction has been given to the patient and the manner in which it has been received. Ideally, you will have the opportunity to personally re-evaluate the patient before termination or expiration of these orders.

Remember that if a patient has displayed violent behavior, placing him or her in a seclusion room without the use of restraints may be inviting disaster. Such patients have been known to bang their heads or throw themselves headlong at the door, sustaining serious injury. This can happen very quickly. If a patient is physically out of control, chemical restraint and/or physical restraint is the safest way to avoid further incident. One-to-one staff observation is also advisable.

Once the patient's safety has been established, further assessment of possible psychiatric and medical causes of the violent behavior can be identified and treated. Be sure to review vital signs taken over the last 48 to 72 hours, and carefully rule out or treat drug or alcohol withdrawal.

If the patient has made specific threats against a particular individual, you are obliged to take the threat seriously. If significant risk of danger to an individual is present, in most jurisdictions you have a duty to inform and take measures to protect that individual before the patient is discharged. In such cases, consult with attending physicians, the hospital risk management and legal team, and/or the ethics committee. Document your concerns and the actions taken clearly and concisely in the chart. Give verbal sign-out of this information to the next physician on duty.

■ REMEMBER

It is your responsibility to help the patient to restore his or her composure in the least restrictive yet safest manner possible. Because it is impossible to assess impulsivity and dangerousness with certainty, take whatever measures are necessary to ensure patient and staff safety.

11 | The Suicidal Patient

KHLEBER CHAPMAN ATTWELL

You will often be called to assess a patient's suicidal ideation. Patients who have just attempted suicide require appropriate emergent medical attention, be it charcoal/gastric lavage, dialysis, or suturing of lacerations, and should be referred as appropriate. Many other avenues of "suicidality" may also present when you are on call: psychiatric inpatients seriously struggling to keep from taking their own lives; intensive care patients looking for a way out of pain; emergency room patients with command auditory hallucinations to kill themselves; or malingerers in search of a sandwich and a cot. Your job becomes discovery of the etiology of the suicidality, provision of the immediate stabilization necessary for safety of the patient, and initiation of appropriate treatment.

■ PHONE CALL

Questions

1. **Has there been a suicide attempt?**
   If so, call the appropriate medical/surgical consultant immediately. If not, determine exactly what the patient said and whether there was a plan. This information will guide the need for a one-to-one suicide protective watch.
2. **Does the patient have a psychiatric history?**
3. **What was the reason for admission?**
4. **Does the patient have any medical problems?**
5. **Does the patient abuse any substances?**
6. **What has the patient's behavior been like on the floor or in the emergency room (ER)?**

Orders

The most important decision to make during the phone call is whether to initiate a one-to-one protective watch immediately, before you arrive to do your evaluation. Typically, the nurse will have spoken to the patient and also may know the patient from the current or a prior stay in the hospital. If the patient has thoughts of suicide but has no current intent to harm himself or herself (and is able to contract for safety [e.g., would approach the staff and ask for help if feelings of impulsivity began to return]), a one-to-one watch generally is not necessary. The agitated, threatening, or bizarre patient, however, will usually benefit from close observation. If unsure, always order the watch and defer the longer term decision about this watch until you have had a chance to perform your entire evaluation. Keep in mind that a patient who might or has harmed himself or herself can just as impulsively harm others under the right circumstances.

Also consider the use of as-needed (PRN) medications. Should the patient prove agitated or extremely anxious, these can be highly effective not only for settling the patient into a more gentle interview but also for minimizing impulsive actions of self-destruction. **Lorazepam 1 to 2 mg** can relieve acute agitation; **2 to 5 mg haloperidol (Haldol)** can dampen intense, frightening auditory hallucinations or acute lability.

Inform RN

"Will arrive in . . . minutes."

As suicidality constitutes a genuinely acute emergency, do everything in your capacity to see the patient immediately.

■ ELEVATOR THOUGHTS

What causes suicidality?
- Major depression (with or without psychotic features)
- Depression not otherwise specified (NOS)
- Adjustment disorders
- Cyclothymic disorders
- Bipolar disorders I and II
- Mood disorders due to general medical conditions
- Schizophrenia
- Schizoaffective disorder
- Alcohol or drug abuse/dependence
- Anxiety disorder (generalized, panic, post-traumatic, obsessive-compulsive)
- Severe personality disorders, particularly borderline personality
- Malingering

■ MAJOR THREAT TO LIFE

A patient who is threatening suicide and has a plan is in a crisis requiring your immediate intervention. Factors that increase risk include age above 45 years, male sex, alcohol dependence, violent behavior, previous suicide attempt, past psychiatric hospitalization, and family history of suicide. Medical illness and social isolation also increase the likelihood of the patient's following through with a plan. Use the initial assessment to survey these factors and to evaluate ways to keep the patient safe.

■ BEDSIDE

Quick Look Test

Does the patient look sad or depressed?

Does he or she show psychomotor agitation or retardation, social withdrawal, and isolation from staff and peers?

Do you suspect, or does the patient complain of, psychotic symptoms?

What does the staff say about the patient's recent appearance, behavior, or presentation in the ER?

Are there any identified triggers?

Is the patient in acute, unmedicated pain?

Has the patient recently been angry, demanding, or manipulative—suggesting substance abuse or personality disorders?

Airway and Vital Signs

Does the patient pose any risk of medical instability—any risk of overdose, altered mental status, or abnormal vital signs?

Chart Review

- Why is the patient in the hospital?
- Does the patient have any medical problems?
- What medications is the patient currently taking, and for how long has the patient been taking them?
- Does the patient have a psychiatric history?
- Does the patient have a substance abuse problem?
- What is the patient's current medical status?
- Has the patient attempted suicide in the past?

Selective History

You have been called because a patient feels suicidal. Talking about suicide may provoke in the patient anxiety (feeling of shame), rage (feelings of being betrayed by concerned family members), or relief (ego-dystonic auditory hallucinations). Initially, it is important that you identify to the patient who you are and why you have been called and ask basic questions about the patient's age and reason for hospitalization. Then, an often successful approach is to follow the patient's lead to a general question about what has been going on recently. Should you find the patient reluctant to talk, try to gain some rapport through an exploration of his or her life and medical histories. Should you find the patient to be floridly thought-disordered or psychotic in other ways, a structured interview may facilitate obtaining the information you most need.

It is often challenging to talk to patients about suicidal thoughts. **It is important to remember that you cannot plant thoughts in the patient's head.** If the patient has a plan, encourage him or her to speak with you about it. Do not, however, put words in the patient's mouth. For example, "Have you thought about how you would kill yourself?" differs from "Would you take an overdose or hang yourself?"

Handle pauses in the interview by waiting. Often moments of silence can provoke anxiety for both the doctor and the patient, but they can also be the moments when the patient weighs and potentially shares his or her most crucial thoughts, making these times potentially valuable points of intervention. Furthermore, if you are comfortable with silence, you may communicate a sense of acceptance to the patient, which in and of itself can be therapeutic.

Focus on the following issues:

- **Recent history:** What has been happening? Have there been any recent stressors, including medical illnesses or untreated pain? Does this time period correlate with an important anniversary or painful event? Is there a sense of hopelessness, guilt, or self-recrimination? Has the patient been feeling sad, blue, or "down in the dumps." Conversely, is there anything the patient enjoys doing? Have there been changes in sleep or appetite? Try to distinguish major depression from dysthymia and adjustment disorders.
- **Suicidal ideation:** Ask the patient about his or her exact thoughts about suicide. How long has the patient been having them? When did they start? Is there more of a wish to be dead than an active plan? If there is a plan, get the details. Does the patient have the means to carry out the plan? (Are there firearms in the home? Are there syringes, catheters, or other hospital supplies at the bedside that might be used in an attempt?) Has the patient thought about what would happen after his or her death? Is there an intent to carry out the plan? If the patient did not follow through with the plan, why not? This question may elicit positive feelings from the patient, for example, about religion or children.

- **Substance abuse:** Is the patient abusing alcohol, cocaine, opiates, benzodiazepines, or other drugs? If so, how much is consumed daily? When did the abuse begin, and when was the last use? You may elicit more information with a question such as "How much do you drink a day?" rather than "Do you drink alcohol?" If the patient actively abuses drugs or alcohol, suicidal ideation may manifest itself as a form of substance-induced mood or withdrawal-induced dysphoria (the latter is particularly relevant in crack cocaine withdrawal).

- **History of suicide attempts or gestures:** As with any history, find out as many details as possible. Did the patient think the attempt would be successful? What treatment was necessary afterward (intubation, dialysis, charcoal/lavage)? Did the patient contact someone in the process (make a phone call after swallowing pills, write a suicide note), or was he or she found by accident? Does the patient regret not having succeeded? Try to determine the nature of the attempt—premeditated with serious attempt versus impulsive versus manipulative.

- **Medical history:** Obtain a thorough medical history, including current health and medications taken. Many patients with untreated postsurgical or other pain may feel suicidal and articulate these thoughts only when expressing relief at being alive once their analgesia has reached an adequate and comfortable level.

- **Past psychiatric history:** Obtain information about previous hospitalizations and treatments. Is there a history of depression, or of a manic episode, especially one with irritable, expansive, grandiose features (e.g., driving at 120 m.p.h. on the interstate and being annoyed at the slowpokes on the road)? Is there any history of psychosis? In addition to lending data for diagnosis, such information may offer insight into the reasons for the suicidal ideation (command auditory hallucinations versus being unable to tolerate the decompensation of one's own mental status versus receiving bizarre messages such as "drink the Drano to eliminate Jupiter in my left ovary").

- **Family and social history:** Is there a family history of psychiatric illness or of suicide? What is the quality of the patient's interpersonal relationships and his or her social safety net? What is the work history, and has there been a recent decline in work habits? Difficulties in these arenas may help clarify the seriousness of the attempt.

- **Parasuicidal history:** Some patients resort to impulsive suicidal types of actions as a way of regulating their internal state. The diagnosis itself may vary widely: antisocial personality, borderline personality, cyclothymia, polysubstance dependence, dependent personality, or malingering. The principle, however, remains the same. These patients present for medical treatment either before or after attempts to harm themselves; these behaviors represent their use of external measures to regulate their internal states. Though usually not lethal, such attempts may become lethal if such patients do not receive attention (by swallowing broken glass instead of pills or actually jumping instead of just threatening to jump). Although these actions are largely impulsive, it is the psychiatrist's job to treat them as psychiatric emergencies until the impulsivity can be contained and treatment recommended.

■ MENTAL STATUS EXAMINATION

A full, current mental status examination is always a vital part of the assessment. Areas of focus include appearance, behavior, lability of mood, and level of psychomotor activity. Is the patient withdrawn, unkempt, or profoundly motorically retarded? Is the speech slowed or pressured? Is the patient sad, anxious, or constricted? Do you feel you could be assaulted at any moment? Does the patient suffer from a thought disorder or from perceptual abnormalities? Are there any auditory hallucinations, particularly command auditory hallucinations? Are they mood congruent? Ask specifically what the voices say and how long they have been heard. Assess suicidal ideation in depth, as discussed earlier. Evaluate the patient's insight and judgment, with particular attention to his or her level of impulsivity.

■ MANAGEMENT

Regardless of the underlying diagnosis, the safety of the patient remains paramount. If the evaluation takes place in the ER, you must decide whether to admit the patient based on your assessment of the current level of risk. You can admit the patient on a voluntary or involuntary basis. Should admission not be indicated, prompt referral for outpatient treatment must follow, including collateral calls to the patient's current outpatient psychiatrist (if he or she has one). If the patient is already admitted to a medical or surgical service and has passive suicidal ideation without intent or plan and is able to contract for safety (e.g., would approach the staff and ask for help if feelings of impulsivity began to return), refer the patient to the hospital's consultation-liaison service for follow-up. If the patient is not at risk to himself or herself, one-to-one observation need not be ordered.

Should the patient be an active risk and unable to contract for safety, initiate a one-to-one watch or transfer the patient to a psychiatric floor. Keep in mind that a one-to-one watch does not begin until the aide is actually at the bedside. Arrange for the aide to arrive as soon as possible, and make sure that the patient is not left alone until the aide does arrive. Avoid at all costs the possibility that a patient may find a way to harm himself or herself between the time the order for the watch is given and the watch actually begins. Always look for methods the patient might use in the immediate vicinity to injure himself or herself.

Treatment starts during the interview. A supportive style, with emphasis on encouraging the patient to share concerns, often proves therapeutic. The patient may benefit from a variety of PRN medications, including trazodone, diphenhydramine, or zolpidem to allow sleep; lorazepam or clonazepam for anxiety; or haloperidol for psychotic symptoms.

In general, starting an antidepressant medication can be deferred until either diagnostic or treatment arrangements have been clarified. Ensure medical clearance to expedite the initiation of pharmacotherapy. Routine tests include complete blood count with differential, electrolytes, liver function tests, thyroid function, rapid plasma reagin for syphilis, electrocardiogram, and urine toxicology.

Table 11–1 □ MEDICAL CONDITIONS ASSOCIATED WITH DEPRESSION

Drugs and toxins: reserpine, alpha-methyldopa, propranolol, cimetidine, steroids

Abused substances: alcohol, cocaine, opiates

Infectious disease: mononucleosis, influenza, viral pneumonia, Lyme borreliosis

Neoplasm: pancreatic cancer, bronchogenic carcinoma, brain tumor, lymphoma

Cardiovascular: hypoxia, mitral valve prolapse

Endocrine: hyperthyroidism, hypothyroidism, hyperparathyroidism, hypoparathyroidism, hyperadrenocortical function, hypoadrenocortical function

Metabolic: uremia, hyponatremia, hypokalemia

Nutritional: pellagra, thiamine deficiency, B_{12} and folate deficiency

Collagen-vascular: systemic lupus erythematosus, rheumatoid arthritis, giant cell arteritis

Central nervous system disease: Parkinson's disease, Huntington's disease, chronic subdural hematoma, temporal lobe epilepsy, stroke

Miscellaneous: Wilson's disease, psoriasis, amyloidosis

Adapted from Ples R: Clinical Manual of Psychiatric Diagnosis and Treatment. Washington, DC, American Psychiatric Press, Inc., 1994, p. 122.

If you believe that the depression at hand stems from a medical illness, discuss this with the treating or consulting internist for follow-up (refer to Table 11–1 for medical considerations). Should you find psychotic symptoms on examination, prescribing an antipsychotic (and discussing with the patient the risks and benefits of typical antipsychotic medications to the extent possible) may facilitate a more rapid recovery. Also consider the patient's prior exposure to antipsychotics, including response and side effects. An appropriate starting point might be **2 to 5 mg haloperidol for an adult patient** who is otherwise healthy and **0.5 to 1 mg for a geriatric patient or a patient with AIDS**.

Should the suicidal ideation stem from substance abuse and/or withdrawal, emergent management and vigilance of vital signs are critical. Use caution when prescribing an anxiolytic or sedative-hypnotic for this type of patient, in order to avoid reviving old pathways of abuse.

Should you believe the suicidality is the result of a personality disorder, assess the need for one-to-one observation and set limits with the patient as to what can be done immediately.

12 | The Psychotic Patient

CHRISTINE DESMOND
SHARON FALCO

Psychosis is a general descriptive term for a phenomenon that may be present in multiple medical and psychiatric conditions. A patient's inability to think, respond emotionally, communicate, perceive and interpret reality, or behave appropriately may be characteristic of psychosis. Psychosis is usually characterized by hallucinations, delusions, impaired reality testing, and sometimes diminished impulse control. Because there are many etiologies for psychosis, your role is to help determine the cause of the psychosis (medical illness, substance- or drug-related, or psychiatric) and to provide a management strategy to the referring physician.

■ PHONE CALL

Questions

1. How is the patient behaving?
2. Is the patient dangerous to himself or herself or to others?
3. What are the reasons for hospitalization?
4. What medications is the patient taking?
5. Have there been any recent changes in level of consciousness?
6. Have there been previous similar episodes?
7. What are the patient's vital signs?

Orders

1. Order the appropriate level of monitoring for the situation. Remember that behavior associated with psychosis is very unpredictable. One-to-one observation may be indicated until you are able to assess the situation personally.
2. In the case of behavior acutely dangerous to either the patient or others, you may verbally order the RN to implement physical restraints or seclusion. Most institutions have their own protocols for restraint and seclusion, as well as for the assistance of hospital security. You should be familiar with these procedures and consider their implementation.

3. At times, psychotic patients may become extremely agitated and will occasionally require as-needed (PRN) medication before they can be safely assessed or in cases of dangerousness.

Inform RN

"Will arrive in . . . minutes."

■ ELEVATOR THOUGHTS

What causes psychosis?

Psychiatric Disorders

- Schizophrenia
- Schizophreniform disorder
- Schizoaffective disorder
- Mood disorders, bipolar disorder, or major depression with psychotic disorders
- Delusional disorder
- Brief reactive psychosis
- Obsessive-compulsive disorder
- Personality disorders
- Psychosis not otherwise specified, postpartum psychosis, or delirium
- Atypical psychosis, autoscopic phenomena, Cotard's syndrome
- Capgras' syndrome
- Malingering
- Factitious disorder

Drug-Induced Psychosis

1. Therapeutic agents
   - Amphetamines
   - Anticholinergic drugs
   - Anticonvulsant drugs
   - Antimalarial drugs
   - Bromides
   - Belladonna alkaloids
   - Cimetidine
   - Steroids
   - Isocarboxizid
   - L-dopa
   - Lidocaine
   - Methylphenidate

- Nitrous oxide
- Phenelzine
- Phenylpropanolamine
- Podophyllin
- Procaine penicillin
- Pyridostigmine
- Sulfonamides

2. Alcohol and illicit drugs
   - Cannabis
   - Cocaine
   - Ethyl alcohol
   - Hallucinogens
   - Phencyclidine
   - Ketamine
   - Other synthesized drugs (e.g., "Ecstasy")

3. Poisoning
   - *Amanita muscaria*
   - Belladonna alkaloids
   - Carbon monoxide

4. Alcohol withdrawal

Medical Conditions (Selected List)

- Acquired immunodeficiency syndrome (AIDS)
- Acute intermittent porphyria
- B_{12} deficiency
- Cerebral lipoidosis
- Creutzfeldt-Jakob disease
- Epilepsy
- Herpes encephalitis
- Homocystinuria
- Huntington's disease
- Hypothyroidism/myxedema
- Neoplasms
- Neurosyphilis
- Normal-pressure hydrocephalus
- Pellagra
- Systemic lupus erythematosus (SLE)
- Wernicke-Korsakoff syndrome

■ MAJOR THREAT TO LIFE

1. Psychosis may be associated with severe medical conditions and may be exacerbated by toxic levels of medications, such as antiarrhythmics, anticonvulsants, or anesthetic agents.
2. Psychotic behavior may result in physical fights, accidents, suicide, or the refusal of treatment.

3. Your role is to prevent harm to other patients and to staff, as well as to implement necessary measures for self-protection.

■ BEDSIDE

Quick Look Test

Does the patient look calm, distressed, or agitated?

Observe the patient's appearance and interaction with family members or caretakers present. Assess posture, grooming, personal hygiene, and clothing. Observe if there is fidgeting, pacing, hyperactivity, tardive dyskinesia, or catatonia. Loud speech, property damage, and combative behavior should be noted. If the patient looks agitated, ask the nursing and medical staff to ensure a safe environment for the patient and others, calling for additional staff and using physical restraints if necessary.

Airway and Vital Signs

What is the heart rate?

Tachycardia may be indicative of withdrawal states or other medical illnesses.

What is the temperature?

Fever may be a sign of sepsis, infection, or neuroleptic malignant syndrome (NMS).

Selective History and Chart Review

Discuss with medical and nursing staff the time course of symptoms and the behavior of the patient as observed. Note the time of onset of any vegetative symptoms, concomitant medical illnesses, and medications taken, including over-the-counter drugs. Obtain a thorough medical history, and note the procedures performed and medications administered. Review old charts for psychiatric history and psychiatric consultations during previous medical hospitalizations. Interview family members or friends accompanying the patient for events leading up to the time of presentation, family history of neurologic or psychiatric illness, and patient's past psychiatric history, including alcohol and drug use.

Selective Physical Examination

A thorough physical examination with special emphasis on the neurologic evaluation should be performed.

Selective Mental Status Examination

- Appearance: poor personal hygiene
- Psychomotor activity: agitation, pacing, combativeness, posturing, stereotyped movements, psychomotor retardation, tremors, perioral movements, restlessness
- Speech: impoverished, mute to mumbling, loud or shouting, pressured
- Affect: inappropriate, labile to constricted, angry, irritable, anxious, depressed or euphoric
- Thought processes: goal directed, coherent or incoherent, looseness of associations, flight of ideas, internal preoccupation, talking to oneself, thought blocking, disorganization, tangentiality, circumstantiality, echolalia, word salad
- Perceptions: hallucinations (visual, auditory, tactile, or olfactory)
- Thought content: paranoia, ideas of reference, magical thinking, delusions of grandiosity or persecution, obsessions or preoccupations, suicidal or homicidal ideation with plan or intent
- Cognitive examination: if level of consciousness, orientation, or memory is impaired, delirium should be suspected.
- Insight and judgment: impaired

Laboratory Evaluation

Review laboratory tests, including routine blood chemistries, liver function tests, electrolytes, VDRL, thyroid function tests, B_{12}, folate, human immunodeficiency virus test, and urinalysis. Urine toxicology tests may also shed light on drug use and withdrawal states. If Wilson's disease is suspected, a serum ceruloplasmin should be drawn. An ophthalmology consultation can be requested for a slit-lamp examination to look for Kayser-Fleischer rings. It may be necessary to perform a computed tomographic (CT) scan of the head and a lumbar puncture (LP) to rule out infectious and neurologic etiologies for an acute onset of psychotic symptoms.

■ MANAGEMENT

Once medical causes are excluded, the determination of dangerousness to the patient or others is the priority in psychiatric disorders. The need to provide a safe and controlled environment with supportive staff is indicated in order to prevent harm or injury to the patient. Appropriate medication includes an antipsychotic, such as **haloperidol (Haldol) 5 mg orally (PO) twice a day (BID),** for initial maintenance. In the case of severe agitation,

haloperidol 5 mg intramuscularly (IM) and repeated every 30 minutes may be necessary to control extreme agitation associated with the psychosis. (Remember that antipsychotic medications tend to lower seizure threshold.) **Lorazepam (Ativan) 2 mg IM and repeated every 30 minutes** may also be necessary, in addition to haloperidol, for a more sedating effect. Administration of **benztropine 1 mg PO BID** or **diphenhydramine 25 mg BID** may provide adequate prophylactic measures against an acute dystonic reaction and should be given if there is a known history of dystonia. Monitoring with frequent observation (i.e., one-to-one watch or checks every 15 minutes) and communication with limit setting during this time will aid in controlling agitation. Consider a change in environment (e.g., go to the patient's room or to a quiet room).

Medical and neurologic disorders should be referred to the appropriate consulting team. Treatment of the underlying etiology of psychosis will eventually lead to clearance of the psychotic symptoms. Treatment with haloperidol may vary from 0.5 mg PO at bedtime for the elderly to 5 to 10 mg PO BID or three times a day (TID) for an average-sized adult. Pregnant patients with chronic psychotic illness may need low maintenance doses of haloperidol rather than benzodiazepines, which should be avoided because of teratogenic effects.

13 | The Confused Patient: Delirium and Dementia

CERI E. HADDA

A patient's confusion in the general medical setting is most often a result of delirium or dementia. Delirium indicates the presence of an acute underlying medical problem (or combination of problems). Less commonly, confusion may be due to conditions such as pseudodementia and amnestic syndrome. Thus, it is important to distinguish between delirium and dementia in order to initiate appropriate medical treatment while trying to reduce the anxiety and agitation often associated with the confusion. Remember that delirium and dementia can appear in the same patient and that demented patients are especially susceptible to delirium. When in doubt, it is always prudent to begin a work-up for delirium because delayed medical treatment may lead to increased morbidity or even mortality, as well as longer hospital stays.

■ DEFINITIONS

Delirium

Delirium is an acute process that heralds medical problems, particularly in elderly, brain-injured, or acutely ill patients, as well as in children. It is characterized by rapid onset, although sometimes the patient will show prodromal behavioral disturbances up to several days before frank delirium sets in. These can include irritability, anxiety, and sleep disturbances.

Delirium usually has a fluctuating course ("waxing and waning"), ranging from clouding of consciousness to coma interrupted by lucid intervals. Typically, symptoms of delirium worsen at night. Disturbances of the sleep-wake cycle and an increased or decreased level of psychomotor activity are hallmarks of the disorder, but features vary widely, frequently making the diagnosis more difficult.

Global impairment of cognition occurs, causing disturbances in memory, perception, and thinking. Delirious patients often have a reduced ability to remain focused, leading to easy distractibility. They may demonstrate disorganized thinking, incoherent speech, and sensory misperceptions, especially visual hallucinations and illusions.

The delirious patient can be either agitated or apathetic, reflecting psychomotor agitation or retardation. Patients may be restless, pick at their bedclothes (floccillation), or try to get out of bed. The physician on call is much more likely to be called for a delirious patient who is combative and agitated, while the "quietly" delirious patient may be overlooked or regarded as depressed and withdrawn.

Emotional disturbances appear in the form of depressed mood, anxiety or fear, paranoia, irritability, euphoria, or apathy. Lability of affect is manifested by rapid shifts between crying, laughter, fear, and anger. Thus, if a patient is described as confused or disoriented, especially with concomitant flux in mood or behavior, delirium is a likely diagnosis.

Sympathetic hyperactivity may occur, including tachycardia, diaphoresis, flushed face, dilated pupils, and elevated blood pressure.

Dementia

Dementia is the decline of higher cortical functions, especially memory, thinking, orientation, comprehension, calculation, learning capacity, language, and judgment. The dysfunction is sufficient to impair activities of daily living and social activities. Although it can occur at any age, dementia is most common in the elderly.

Unlike in delirium, consciousness is typically clear in dementia (i.e., the patient is alert). Depending on the etiology, dementia may have a sudden or insidious onset, be progressive with a long duration, be static, or have a remitting course.

Primary symptoms of dementia include memory loss, particularly difficulty in learning new information (immediate memory), recalling recent events (recent memory), and remembering past personal information (remote memory). Impairment in abstract thinking, judgment, and impulse control; neglect of personal appearance and hygiene; personality changes, anxiety, or depression; paranoid ideation; and irritability are all associated with dementia.

Pseudodementia

Pseudodementia is a severe type of major depression with symptoms similar to dementia, such as withdrawal, decline in concrete thinking, and loss of memory. History of a previous mood disorder, recent emotional distress, and loss of short-term and long-term memory may help distinguish pseudodementia from dementia.

Amnestic Disorder

Amnestic disorder is characterized by memory impairment with no other cognitive deficits that affect occupational or social functioning. Because amnesia may have psychologic or organic etiologies, it is important to take a careful history. Electroconvulsive therapy (ECT), psychologic stress, or a recent traumatic event all may contribute to amnesia.

■ PHONE CALL

Questions

1. How old is the patient?
2. Is the patient agitated or a threat to himself or herself or to others?
3. Is this an acute mental status change?
4. What is the level of consciousness or agitation?
5. What are the vital signs?
6. Are there any associated symptoms or signs (e.g., chest pain, hallucinations, jaundice, or tremors)?
7. What is the patient's diagnosis or reason for admission?
8. Have there been previous episodes of confusion?
9. What is the medical history?
10. What medications is the patient taking? Have any new medications been added or discontinued? Has there been a change in dosage or scheduling?
11. Does the patient abuse alcohol or drugs? When was the last known use?

Orders

1. Ask the staff to provide one-to-one observation if the patient is dangerous to himself or herself or to others.
2. Restraints can be applied if absolutely necessary.
3. Medication can be administered if indicated (e.g., haloperidol for psychotic agitation), but you should see the patient before prescribing medication whenever possible.

Inform RN

"Will arrive in . . . minutes."

■ ELEVATOR THOUGHTS

What causes confusion?

Delirium

Potential causes of delirium are many. They can be roughly divided into those due to chronic cerebral disease, such as dementia, systemic illness, or recreational drug or medication toxicity, and those due to drug or medication withdrawal. Sometimes the cause may be a combination of these disturbances.

Generally the most common causes of delirium are the following:

- Hypoglycemia or marked hyperglycemia
- Fever
- Alcohol withdrawal
- Drug reaction or intoxication
- Polypharmacy (and drug interactions), including use of over-the-counter medications
- Head trauma
- Recent surgery, especially involving general anesthesia

The most common causes found in patients at various sites in the hospital are the following:

- **Emergency room:** head trauma, drug intoxication, cerebro-vascular accidents
- **Medical, surgical, and intensive care units:** fever, electrolyte imbalance, sepsis, alcohol withdrawal, postoperative states, hypoglycemia, medication, polypharmacy, urinary tract infections
- **Psychiatric units:** medication, drug intoxication, alcohol withdrawal, depression, catatonia, fever

Dementia

The most common causes of confusion linked to dementia are the following:

- **Alzheimer's disease:** The number one cause of dementia, Alzheimer's disease has an insidious onset with progressive decline in functioning.
- **Multi-infarct dementia:** The second leading cause of dementia, multi-infarct dementia presents more acutely with an incremental stepwise loss of function. The medical conditions leading to multi-infarct dementia, such as diabetes, hypertension, cardiac disease, and embolic disease from prosthetic valves, may be controlled to prevent further episodes of infarct that may lead to progression of the dementia.

Other causes include

- Brain injury (especially chronic subdural hematoma)
- Central nervous system infections, including human immunodeficiency virus (HIV), neurosyphilis, and tubercular and fungal infections (meningitis, viral encephalitis)
- Pernicious anemia
- Folic acid deficiency
- Bromide intoxication
- Normal-pressure hydrocephalus
- Huntington's chorea

- Multiple sclerosis
- Pick's disease
- Parkinson's disease
- Creutzfeldt-Jacob disease
- Cerebellar degeneration
- Postanoxic or posthypoglycemic states
- Lewey body dementia

Pseudodementia

In the setting of major depression, a patient may also present as confused. In this context, a presentation of confusion is known as pseudodementia.

Amnestic Disorder

If the confusion appears due to an amnestic disorder, consider the following in the differential diagnosis:

- Head trauma or neurologic signs may indicate a brain tumor, a cerebrovascular accident, or seizures.
- Alcoholism is a common cause of blackouts, seizures, or vitamin deficiencies (Korsakoff's syndrome).
- Wernicke's encephalopathy may be revealed by the triad of ophthalmoplegia, ataxia, and delirium.
- Psychogenic amnesia may arise as a defense or for secondary gain. Immediate recall and anterograde memory usually are not affected.
- Psychogenic fugue, associated with alcoholism, involves loss of personal identity and/or remote memory.

■ MAJOR THREAT TO LIFE LEADING TO DELIRIUM

Although delirium secondary to any cause is a medical emergency, some causes are potentially life threatening. They include the following:

- Intracranial hemorrhage
- Sepsis
- Shock
- Narcotic overdose
- Intracranial neoplasm
- Delirium tremens (alcohol withdrawal)
- Arrhythmias

■ REMEMBER

Frequently, an extensive work-up for delirium will not yield a definitive medical cause. Nonetheless, delirium is a clinical diagnosis, indicating one or more causes leading to brain dysfunction; these causes need not be identified in order to make a diagnosis of delirium.

■ BEDSIDE

Quick Look Test

Does the patient look calm, distressed, or agitated?
Observe the patient's appearance and interaction with others. If the patient is agitated, ask the staff to ensure a safe environment, using restraints if necessary.

Airway and Vital Signs

What is the patient's heart rate?
Tachycardia may be indicative of withdrawal states or other medical illnesses.

What is the patient's blood pressure?
Hypertensive encephalopathy and hypotension from blood loss may lead to mental status changes. Hypertension may also be indicative of alcohol withdrawal.

What is the patient's temperature?
Fever may be a sign of sepsis or infection.

What is the patient's respiratory rate?
A rapid respiratory rate may indicate hypoxia secondary to pulmonary embolus or compromised pulmonary function.

Selective History and Chart Review

What is the history of this episode of confusion?
Ask staff about the time course and whether it has been episodic or continuous.

What preceded the episode?
Obtain a thorough medical history, and note procedures and medications before the onset of confusion. Review the medication record to rule out errors in transcription or administration of as-needed (PRN) medication.

What do the nursing notes reveal?
Review the nursing notes for documentation of a change in the patient's mental status, difficulty at night (sundowning), or the fluctuating nature of agitation or confusion.

Were there earlier psychiatric consultations?

Review old charts from previous hospitalizations to assess the patient's behavior in similar settings and situations.

What do friends and family know?

Interview those available as to observed changes in the patient before hospitalization.

Selective Physical Examination

Perform a thorough physical examination, with special emphasis on the neurologic component, to rule out underlying medical illness.

■ DELIRIUM

Selective Mental Status Examination

- A fluctuating level of consciousness may be noted as confusion alternating with lucidity or agitation alternating with stupor.
- Psychomotor activity may include combativeness, picking at sheets, or drifting to sleep during the interview.
- Speech may be mumbling, normal, or shouting.
- Thought processes may be incoherent, rambling, or disorganized.
- Altered perceptual states may be present, including hallucinations (visual, auditory, tactile, olfactory), paranoia, and illusions or delusions regarding procedures or staff.
- Anxiety, irritability, depression or euphoria, nightmares, and insomnia with disorientation may occur.
- Sundowning is typical in the elderly and is characterized by disorientation at night, falls, wandering, illusions, or hallucinations.

Laboratory Tests

An array of tests may be necessary to isolate the underlying cause or causes of the confusion. These should include a complete blood count with differential; liver function tests; electrolytes; erythrocyte sedimentation rate (remember that elderly patients normally have higher levels); Venereal Disease Research Laboratory test (VDRL) for syphilis; thyroid function tests (measure thyroid-stimulating hormone [TSH] level first); HIV test; arterial blood gases; and urinalysis.

If fever is present, urinalysis and urine and blood cultures may reveal the source of the infection causing the fever. A chest x-ray (CXR) may reveal pneumonia.

Urine and/or serum drug toxicology tests may reveal drug use or withdrawal. A head computed tomography (CT) scan and/or lumbar puncture (LP) may be needed to rule out infectious or neurologic causes for an acute change in mental status.

Management

Structured Environment

Delirium is potentially reversible with treatment of the underlying medical disorder. In the interim, provide a safe and structured environment to limit harm to the patient or to others. If possible, the patient should be moved to a room where he or she will not be isolated and can be easily monitored. Staff should provide repeated explanations of procedures and tests, as well as clocks and calendars, to keep the patient oriented. The presence of family members and familiar objects is also reassuring to the patient.

Treatment of the Underlying Medical Disorder

Medication-Related Delirium. Medications are implicated in up to 30% of cases of delirium. Although almost any drug can contribute to delirium in susceptible individuals, certain categories of medications frequently lead to acute and even chronic confusional states.

Drugs with known anticholinergic properties include long-acting benzodiazepines, opioids, tricyclic antidepressants, and some of the older antihypertensive medications such as reserpine and clonidine. In addition, H_2 blockers, other cardiac medications such as digoxin, nonsteroidal anti-inflammatory drugs (NSAIDs), antibiotics, and corticosteroids have been determined to contribute to delirium in the susceptible individual.

Treatment of medication-related delirium involves discontinuing the responsible medication(s). To reduce the likelihood of adverse reaction, heed the adage, "start low and go slow."

Other Underlying Problems
- **Hypoxia, metabolic disorders, and endocrine abnormalities:** Treatment of hypoxia, metabolic disorders, and endocrine abnormalities can often quickly clear delirium.
- **Infections:** Infection leading to delirium can be as simple as a urinary tract infection in an elderly patient.
- **Postoperative status:** Whether due to general anesthesia or an underlying medical complication, delirium is often found in the postoperative patient.
- **Toxins:** Toxicologic tests may shed light on drug use and withdrawal states.
- **"ICU psychosis":** Intensive care unit (ICU) psychosis is a

misnomer for a delirium that is associated with agitation in an intensive care setting. Control of the agitation in a timely manner is a priority, as are attempts to understand what may be contributing to the patient's delirium.

Medications to Treat the Underlying Disorder. As stated earlier, the most important treatment for delirium is determining and trying to eliminate the medical problem or problems leading to the syndrome. Therefore, any necessary medication changes toward that end, such as beginning antibiotics, lowering dosages, or changing maintenance medications, must be initiated.

Calming the Delirious Patient.   Haloperidol (Haldol) with or without lorazepam (Ativan) is useful for calming the agitated, paranoid, or belligerent patient. Care must be taken to avoid respiratory suppression with lorazepam. **Haloperidol should be administered 1 to 5 mg by mouth (PO) or intramuscularly (IM),** and may be repeated several times every 30 minutes if agitation persists. Haloperidol and lorazepam may be administered together intravenously, at dosages of **haloperidol 0.5 to 5 mg** and **lorazepam 1 to 2 mg** as an initial dose. Dosing may be repeated several times every 30 minutes if agitation has not been controlled.

Both elderly and brain-injured patients should be treated with lower amounts of the medications to begin with. The drugs may be titrated upward as warranted.

When intravenous (IV) haloperidol is used, the patient's cardiac status should be carefully monitored, because cases of torsades de pointes have been reported with the use of IV haloperidol.

Physical restraints should be avoided unless there is a threat to the patient's safety, the safety of others, or the integrity of the IV lines, tubes, or other connections.

■ DEMENTIA

Selective Mental Status Examination

- Cognitive changes are notable over time, with loss of date, time, and memory for recent events occurring first, followed by loss of place and then person.
- Learning new tasks may become impossible, followed by the inability to perform activities of daily living (ADLs).
- Aphasia, agnosia, and apraxia may be evident.
- Loss of abstract thinking and judgment may lead to poor impulse control, indiscretions, and violations of social norms.
- Affect may be labile with changes in personality.
- Denial, angry outbursts, or anxiety may be present.

- The patient may exhibit depression or psychosis with paranoia or delusions.
- Psychomotor activity may be characterized by agitation, assaultive behavior, withdrawal, or retardation.

Remember that the mini-mental status examination is not diagnostic, but it can be used over a period of time to follow progression of dysfunction.

Laboratory Tests

To help clarify the patient's diagnosis, additional tests for dementia may include blood chemistries and measurements of vitamin B_{12}, folate, and heavy metal levels. Nutritional deficiencies have also been identified as causative in some patients with dementia.

Management

Dementia is a disorder of brain function and cognition. It is occasionally reversible. Even when its progression is inevitable, steps may be taken to manage certain signs and symptoms that are distressing to the patient, his or her family, and staff caring for the patient.

Behavioral therapy, reality orientation, and environmental manipulations are three frequently used management techniques.

Depression in the context of dementia symptoms may be the result of pseudodementia or it may be a mood disorder superimposed on true dementia. Cognitive dysfunction with pseudodementia can be expected to resolve with successful treatment of the depression, whereas it will persist in the demented patient even when the depression is successfully treated.

Treatment of the Underlying Medical Disorder

In some forms of dementia, treating the underlying cause will often reverse the disorder. Some underlying causes include the following:

- Some nutritional deficiencies may cause dementia; supplement by adding nutrients to the daily regimen.
- A history of drug and alcohol abuse may reveal delirium tremens (DTs) or sedative-hypnotic withdrawal.
- Subdural hematoma may be associated with a history of trauma or frequent falls.
- Normal-pressure hydrocephalus may be diagnosed with the triad of dementia, incontinence, and gait apraxia. Obtain a neurology consult if this disorder is suspected.
- Intracranial masses and lesions may be seen on head CT scan.
- Encephalitis, tertiary syphilis, and fungal meningitis may be revealed by LP.

- Pseudodementia is associated with a normal electroencephalogram (EEG); true dementia is not.

Medications

Superimposed psychiatric symptoms in the elderly demented patient may be targeted with medications. Anticholinergic agents and benzodiazepines should be avoided, secondary to the risk of delirium in the elderly.

Psychotropic medications in the elderly and brain-impaired should be initiated at one third to one half of the usual adult dose. They can be slowly titrated upward as clinically warranted to minimize side effects.

Psychosis may be treated with atypical antipsychotics such as risperidone or olanzapine, which are associated with a lower likelihood of the tardive dyskinesia and extrapyramidal side effects to which elderly individuals are particularly susceptible. **Haloperidol** may also be used **IM or PO at 0.5 to 1.0 mg at bedtime (QHS) or twice a day (BID).**

Insomnia may be treated with **trazodone (Desyrel) 25 to 50 mg PO QHS.** As with other anticholinergics, diphenhydramine (Benadryl) should be avoided.

■ AMNESIA

Selective Mental Status Examination

Common manifestations include the following:
- Loss of memory
- Retrograde, anterograde, circumscribed amnesia
- Confabulation
- Denial
- Apathy

Management

1. Treatment of the underlying medical disorder should resolve the amnestic disorder.
2. An amobarbital sodium interview or hypnosis may be indicated for psychogenic amnesia or fugue.

14 | Rigidity and Neuroleptic Malignant Syndrome

ADAM RAFF

Frequently one may be called to evaluate a patient's complaint of feeling stiff or to observe clinically his or her rigidity. The causes may vary, and the clinician should be equipped to distinguish commonly encountered or reversible problems (e.g., acute dystonia, drug-induced parkinsonism) from more lethal conditions, namely, neuroleptic malignant syndrome (NMS). While the more common problems represent some of the most dramatic presentations in the field of psychiatry, they can be treated rapidly, effectively, and easily. In contrast, NMS represents one of the few life-threatening psychiatric emergencies that require close scrutiny in diagnosis and management in order to minimize high mortality rates. NMS inevitably entails transfer of the patient to an intensive care unit.

■ PHONE CALL

Questions

1. Are there any other associated signs or symptoms such as fever, muscle spasms, difficulty breathing, diaphoresis, dysphagia, drooling, or tremor?
2. What are the current and recent vital signs? What is the level of consciousness?
3. Are there any acute or chronic medical problems?
4. Is the patient taking or has there been a recent addition of an antipsychotic medication to the medication regimen?
5. When did the rigidity begin? Is it generalized, or is it only in certain body areas?
6. Was the onset sudden or gradual?

Orders

1. When triaging responsibilities, one must pay immediate and careful attention to the reports of rigidity in the context of vital sign abnormalities (particularly fever), difficulties in respiration, and changes in mental status. In cases of suspected NMS, ask the nurse to hold all medications until you arrive and examine the patient.

2. In cases of suspected acute dystonia, ask the nurse to prepare **benztropine 1 to 2 mg intramuscularly (IM)** or **diphenhydramine 25 to 50 mg IM** before your arrival. For milder cases of dystonia, you may either wait until you examine the patient or ask the nurse to prepare the above medications in oral (PO) form.
3. If you are unable to see the dystonic patient immediately and you order these medications, be sure to follow up on the patient's response. If there is no significant change, you must examine the patient as soon as possible.

Inform RN

"Will arrive in . . . minutes."

■ ELEVATOR THOUGHTS

What are causes of rigidity?

Neuroleptic Malignant Syndrome

- NMS is characterized by rigidity, hyperthermia, mental status changes, elevated creatine kinase (CK) level, and autonomic instability.
- NMS is rare but life threatening, with mortality rates of 20%.
- Transfer to intensive medical care should be immediate.
- In cases of mild to moderate temperature elevations with variable rigidity, be sure to consider the medication and substance abuse history in order to rule out other toxic syndromes (anticholinergic-related or monoamine oxidase inhibitor [MAOI]-related serotonin syndromes). As well, rule out infections (e.g., meningitis), metabolic defects, malignant hyperthermia, heat stroke, myocardial infarction, drug allergies and side effects, drug interactions, and lethal catatonia.

Acute Dystonia

- Acute dystonia is characterized by sustained muscular spasms or contractions.
- It is easily reversible with antiparkinsonian or antihistaminic agents.
- Laryngeal involvement can be life threatening and may be characterized by dyspnea or subjective respiratory distress.
- Onset often follows recent administration of an antipsychotic.
- Rule out other possible causes such as metabolic defects, central nervous disorders, tumors, head trauma, and toxins.
- Nonpsychiatric medications that have been associated with

dystonia include antiemetics, toxic levels of phenytoin, levo-dopa, and antimalarials containing quinine.
- Anxiety can exacerbate the worsening condition.

Drug-Induced Parkinsonism

- Drug-induced parkinsonism is characterized by rigidity, resting tremor, bradykinesia, and stooped posture, which are clinically identical to the symptoms of idiopathic parkinsonism.
- Onset is often within several weeks of antipsychotic administration or change.
- Antipsychotic medications are the most likely causative agents.
- Rule out other possible causes, such as degenerative central nervous system (CNS) diseases, metabolic defects, brain tumors, head injuries, infectious agents, vascular abnormalities, and toxins.
- Rule out idiopathic Parkinson's disease, which, in an elderly patient, may already be an underlying condition.

■ MAJOR THREAT TO LIFE

- NMS
- Laryngeal dystonia

■ BEDSIDE

Quick Look Test

Assess the patient for signs and symptoms consistent with either NMS or laryngeal dystonia. In addition to difficulty breathing, the patient may have problems speaking owing to involvement of pharyngeal musculature. Does the patient appear toxic and or dehydrated? Although very uncomfortable, patients with milder forms of dystonia and drug-induced parkinsonism may continue to follow their daily routines before asking for help. Conversely, patients with suspected NMS are frequently bedridden and dehydrated and appear quite sick.

Airway and Vital Signs

Most antipsychotic-induced conditions that produce rigidity do not compromise the autonomic system, except for NMS and laryngeal dystonia. In NMS, there usually is a significant elevation in temperature accompanied by tachycardia, tachypnea, and either hypertension or hypotension.

■ NEUROLEPTIC MALIGNANT SYNDROME

Neuroleptic malignant syndrome is a rare but potentially fatal illness. It occurs in about 0.2% of patients treated with antipsychotics. A wide range of signs and symptoms are associated with NMS.

Selective Physical Examination

Look for the following signs (which often evolve in this sequence):

1. Mental status changes
2. Rigidity (lead-pipe or cogwheel)
3. Hyperthermia
4. Autonomic dysfunction

Some patients have a variant of NMS in which only two or three of these features are present. Symptoms of autonomic dysfunction range from rapid and irregular heart rates and hypertension to tachypnea, diaphoresis, and urinary incontinence. Also pay attention to

- Dysphagia, dysarthria, sialorrhea
- Akinesia, bradykinesia, tremor
- Fluctuating level of awareness

The patient initially may be quite alert but may later become agitated or obtunded. Other neurologic features such as seizures, ataxia, and nystagmus can eventually develop.

Laboratory Findings

While NMS must always be considered in complaints of rigidity, it is also a diagnosis of exclusion. Other disorders must first be ruled out, especially in the context of abnormal laboratory values. There are no pathognomonic laboratory findings in NMS, but certain abnormalities may support the diagnosis:

1. Elevated levels of CK are most frequently noted in NMS. They indicate prolonged muscle contraction and trauma. Elevations can be either minimal or exceed 100,000.
2. The white blood cell count may be increased secondary to hyperthermia and mounting muscular inflammation.
3. Aldolase, alkaline phosphatase, serum aspartate transaminase (AST), and serum alanine transaminase (ALT) may be elevated.
4. Blood serum levels of calcium, iron, and magnesium may be decreased.
5. Proteinuria and myoglobinuria may be present. Acute renal failure is a common complication of NMS due to the buildup and overwhelming burden of proteins from muscle breakdown.

Physical Examination

- Conduct careful medical, neurologic, and mental status examinations. Be aware of the four major features of NMS: rigidity, hyperthermia, autonomic instability, and mental status changes.
- Palpate the skull for evidence of head trauma.
- Check the size and symmetry of the pupils. Pinpoint pupils suggest narcotic abuse; dilated pupils suggest sympathomimetic abuse.
- Examine the neck for nuchal rigidity (meningitis).
- Auscultate the heart for new murmurs (endocarditis).
- Listen to the lungs to rule out any signs indicating respiratory tract infection.
- Palpate the abdomen for tenderness (surgical abdomen).
- Examine for any skin rashes (drug reactions, infections).
- In the mental status examination, be sure to focus on appearance, degree of alertness, level of consciousness, affect, perceptual or thought distortions, and any other motor abnormalities.
- In the neurologic examination, note any focal findings, rigidity, or tremors.

Management

If the patient has been taking an antipsychotic and you cannot identify a specific cause for the rigidity (e.g., infection), you must entertain the possibility that your patient is developing NMS. It is crucial for the clinician to recognize NMS so that both supportive and dopaminergic therapies can be instituted before the onset of irreversible complications.

1. Discontinue the antipsychotic medication.
2. Order the required laboratory tests, including a complete blood count, electrolytes, urinanalysis, CK, alkaline phosphatase, SGOT, SGPT, and full fever work-up.
3. Call in a medical or neurologic consultant.
4. Arrange a bed in the intensive care unit.
5. Provide supportive care for fever (e.g., intravenous [IV] hydration, cooling blankets, ice baths).
6. Consider initiating treatment with dantrolene sodium or bromocriptine, the most commonly used medications to treat patients with NMS.
   - Dantrolene sodium is a skeletal muscle relaxant that can be given parenterally or orally. It lessens the muscle rigidity and hyperthermia. (There are studies to suggest that reversal of the rigidity correlates with resolution of autonomic instability.) **The recommended dosage of dantrolene is 2 to 3 mg/kg IV four times a day. The total daily**

IV dose is about 10 mg/kg; hepatotoxicity is associated with higher dosages. **The suggested oral dose ranges from 50 to 600 mg daily.**

- Bromocriptine is a dopaminergic agonist. It is the treatment of choice for patients who can tolerate oral medications. Patients are started on **2.5 to 5 mg PO three times per day (TID).** The dose is then increased by **2.5 mg TID every 24 hours** until the patient begins to respond. **The maximum daily dose is 60 mg.** It should be noted that bromocriptine can exacerbate or cause psychosis. The length of treatment with dantrolene, bromocriptine, or both depends on the form of the antipsychotic that caused the NMS. For patients taking oral antipsychotics, a course of 10 days' treatment is necessary, whereas those patients taking depot antipsychotics (e.g., Haldol Decanoate) require up to 2 to 3 weeks of treatment.

Remember

The clinical course of NMS is variable but usually progresses rapidly. About 40% of patients go on to develop medical complications involving the respiratory system (e.g., aspiration pneumonia) or the cardiovascular, renal, or nervous system. The mortality rate can be as high as 20%. NMS often develops within the first few days of treatment with an antipsychotic or after its dosage is increased. It can also emerge unexpectedly in a patient who has been taking medication for some time. Risk factors include hypersensitivity to dopaminergic agents, co-morbid affective disorders, and physical illness (e.g., dehydration). High-potency antipsychotics, large dosages, rapid dosage increases within a brief span of time, and parenteral administration are also risk factors. There is mounting evidence to suggest that the use of atypical antipsychotics (e.g., clozapine) may lower the risk of developing NMS.

■ ACUTE DYSTONIA

Acute dystonia is a common movement disorder in patients treated with antipsychotics. It is characterized by muscle spasms and contractions that result in a variety of abnormal postures. Patients usually develop drug-induced dystonia within days of beginning treatment or of having a significant dosage increase. Signs of dystonia may appear or be reported in a discontinuous pattern, with the patient periodically noting discomfort and spasm with transient resolution. Its manifestations can be localized to a single part of the body or may be segmental, involving multiple muscular groups. The movements initially may be sporadic and tremor-like, before developing into the final form of contraction. The following are some other manifestations of antipsychotic-induced acute dystonia:

1. Protruding tongue, difficulty swallowing, mouths tightly shut with various grimaces
2. Torticollis (head twisted to one side)
3. Retrocollis (head forced directly backward)
4. Oculogyric crises (eyes rolled upward, sometimes laterally)
5. Laryngopharyngeal spasms (affected patients experience a feeling of suffocation; laryngeal dystonia may cause sudden death)

Physical Examination

Conduct a complete neurologic examination, observing for common signs of acute dystonia. Patients with laryngeal dystonia will often have audible or auscultated stridor on examination.

Management

1. For laryngeal dystonia, administer **benztropine 2 mg IV or IM stat.** If necessary, you may give another dose in 5 to 10 minutes. In cases of incomplete resolution, give **lorazepam 1 to 2 mg IV/IM slowly.**
2. For severe (nonlaryngeal) dystonic reactions, reassure the patient that this is a common and treatable side effect of the antipsychotic. Again, administer an anticholinergic (e.g., **benztropine 1 to 2 mg IM/IV**) or antihistamine (e.g., **diphenhydramine 25 to 50 mg IM/IV**) immediately. You may repeat these dosages twice in 15 minute intervals if there is an absent or limited response. Be prepared to consider other causes for the patient's prolonged muscle spasm.
3. Once the episode has resolved, be sure to place the patient on standing PO dosages of the above medications to prevent further repeated complications. Typical regimens include **diphenhydramine 25 mg PO two to four times per day, trihexyphenidyl 1 to 3 mg PO three times per day,** and **benztropine 1 to 3 mg PO twice per day.**
4. Consider prophylactic medication for patients who are at high risk of developing dystonia.
5. Educate the patient. Dystonia can be a fearful and painful event for someone who has never had the experience. Careful explanations and supportive contact can mollify an already charged situation and even prevent future noncompliance with the antipsychotic medications.

■ DRUG-INDUCED PARKINSONISM

The condition is characterized by muscular rigidity, akinesia (lack of spontaneous motor activity), and tremor, with the former more common than the latter two findings. It usually occurs within the first several days to weeks of antipsychotic initiation. Drug-induced parkinsonism is a more common problem than dystonia, with almost 50% of outpatients developing signs or symptoms during their course of treatment. Unlike patients with drug-induced acute dystonia, however, patients with drug-induced parkinsonism are often unaware that they are experiencing this medication side effect. The clinical features are identical to those associated with idiopathic Parkinson's disease, and its presentation may often worsen the underlying negative symptoms of schizophrenia. Risk factors include older patients, high-potency antipsychotics, and female sex.

Physical Examination

1. Conduct a complete neurologic examination, observing for findings consistent with parkinsonism.
2. Examine the neck, elbows, and wrists for evidence of rigidity. There are two types of rigidity: cogwheel (ratchet-like movements at wrist and elbow) and continuous ("lead-pipe"). Check for cogwheel rigidity at the elbow while having the patient open and close the hand. The severity of rigidity can vary from joint to joint in the same limb.
3. Observe for signs of akinesia, which may manifest as decreased blinking (staring), swallowing (drooling), and spontaneous movements while at rest. There is also a decrease in facial movements (masked facies).
4. Observe for bradykinesia by having the patient tap the fingers together as quickly as possible. Note any tremors. Characteristically, the parkinsonian tremor involves the hands and less commonly the tongue, jaw, and feet. Check for any pill rolling tremors of the fingers.
5. Patients with drug-induced parkinsonism demonstrate postural instability (e.g., retropulsion), and they are often stooped at rest. The gait is characterized by their taking an increasing number of shorter and faster steps (festinating gait).

Management

1. Decrease the antipsychotic dosage if possible.
2. Consider administering a lower-potency antipsychotic as this may decrease the risk of such a side effect.
3. Many patients, particularly the elderly, respond slowly and

incompletely to the use of anticholinergics, antihistamines, and amantadine. Elderly patients are susceptible to cognitive impairment while taking these medications, and therefore these medications should be used sparingly and only as modifications to a change in the antipsychotic regimen. **Benztropine may be given 1 to 2 mg PO twice a day (BID). Amantadine can be started at 100 mg PO BID** and increased to **200 mg PO BID.** If administered, these medications should be tapered at the earliest indication and in a gradual manner. Drug-induced parkinsonism may be exacerbated by abrupt discontinuation.

4. Atypical antipsychotics (serotonin-dopamine antagonists) may represent an alternative medication strategy as they possess a lower risk for extrapyramidal side effects.

15 | Mutism and Other Problems With Speech and Communication

BRIAN D. BRONSON

The on-call evaluation of new changes in speech or communication requires consideration of a broad differential diagnosis. An array of deficits in speech, ranging from dysarthria to complete mutism, must be differentiated from pathology of cerebral language areas as seen in aphasia or delirium. Changes in speech and language may in themselves be caused by a wide array of psychiatric, medical, and neurologic etiologies. Thus, the clinician's first role is to make this distinction so that proper evaluation and treatment may be pursued.

■ PHONE CALL

Questions

1. How specifically has speech or communication changed? Describe it.
2. What is the patient's level of consciousness?
3. What are the patient's psychiatric, medical, and neurologic histories?
4. Are there alterations in vital signs?
5. What is the patient's level of psychomotor activity? Is catatonia suspected?
6. Did the patient recently begin to take an antipsychotic medication?
7. Is there any suspicion of recent illicit drug use?

Orders

Have the RN take full vital signs if not already measured.

Inform RN

"Will arrive in . . . minutes."
Mutism in any suspected case of psychosis, depression, or

mania in a patient unknown to you warrants one-to-one observation pending your arrival.

■ ELEVATOR THOUGHTS

What causes an acute change in speech or communication?

Mutism is a neuropsychiatric symptom, not a disease. It is a cessation of speech production and attempts at speech production, despite normal alertness, intact cerebral language centers, and intact vocal/oral mechanisms of speech. It may occur in isolation but commonly exists as part of catatonia. Common psychiatric etiologies of mutism include schizophrenia, mania, depression, conversion disorders, malingering, and brief dissociative episodes. Acute medication or drug intoxication states may cause mutism (see later). Many medical etiologies may also cause mutism. Complete mutism should be differentiated from selective mutism, generally seen in children but also seen in depression and paranoid states.

Aphasias are disorders of language. Severely affected patients may present with a near-total inability to produce verbal language, mimicking mutism. Alternatively, an aphasia that impairs language comprehension may rarely mimic psychotic thought disorders. Aphasias typically result from lesions, usually vascular infarcts, in the left cerebral hemisphere.

Dysarthria is a deficit specifically in articulation. It is caused by problems of the neuromusculature of the mouth, lips, or tongue or of the cerebral or cerebellar structures that coordinate their control. It may appear as slurred speech or as a total inability to speak in extensive cases. Note also that dysarthria may be caused specifically by antipsychotic medications. A disorder of phonation, or **dysphonia,** stems from pathology of the larynx.

Altered language in the context of a confusional state requires a work-up for **delirium.**

■ MAJOR THREAT TO LIFE

- Inadequate nutrition from catatonia
- Disordered language from delirium, particularly with deteriorating vital signs
- Mutism in neuroleptic malignant syndrome (NMS)
- Aphasia from acutely evolving stroke
- Agitation, paranoia, violence, and suicidality in severe sensory aphasia
- Violent behavior of psychotic or manic patients coming out of catatonia

- Suicide in severely depressed patients coming out of catatonia

■ BEDSIDE

Quick Look Test

What is the patient's age?

Older patients with any new, acute communication deficit require evaluation for stroke and delirium. In children, loss of speech is typically from selective mutism, a treatable, non–life-threatening condition. In young and middle-aged adults, new-onset mutism is more frequently caused by psychiatric disorders; however, drug and medication toxicity, as well as metabolic disturbances, warrant consideration.

What is the patient's level of consciousness?

Impaired arousal or alertness suggests medical or neurologic etiology. Consider stroke as well as toxic and metabolic causes of delirium, including NMS. Visible diaphoresis or tremor may suggest delirium tremens from alcohol, benzodiazepine, or barbiturate withdrawal.

What is the level of psychomotor activity?

An alert patient with a "frozen" or bizarre posture may have mutism in catatonia (see later). Catatonia may derive from multiple psychiatric and neurologic etiologies.

What is the patient's level of distress?

Patients with mutism from psychiatric causes generally do not appear distressed by their communication deficit. Similarly, patients with amotivational states from frontal lobe pathology are less distressed. However, patients with aphasias, particularly motor aphasias (see later), are quite distressed.

Is the patient breathing comfortably?

Irregular (Cheyne-Stokes) respiration may point to a neurologic cause such as cerebral embolism or infarct.

Does the patient have a new unilateral facial droop?

New-onset changes in speech with a new facial droop point toward ongoing cerebral ischemia or infarct and require immediate neurologic consultation.

Are there any abnormalities in vital signs?

Unstable vital signs may indicate cerebral infarction, drug (illicit or prescribed) intoxication or withdrawal, metabolic derangements, epilepsy, anoxia, infection, or other medical etiologies.

Selective History and Chart Review

Often a full history is not obtainable from the patient. Family members or close friends may provide a history of prior changes in speech; psychiatric, medical, or neurologic illness; or use of medications or illicit drugs. Prior hospital records are also quite useful. Additionally, some patients may be able to write or whisper information.

Has the onset of the change in speech been sudden or gradual?
Gradual loss of verbal communication may be caused by progressive degenerative brain disease (Alzheimer's dementia, frontal-temporal dementia, primary progressive aphasia, Parkinson's disease), neoplasm, or depression. Alternatively, aphasia from stroke typically evolves within hours to days. Traumatic brain injury, delirium, and some psychiatric disorders may also cause more acute changes in communication.

Does the patient have a psychiatric history?
Is there a prior history of mutism or catatonia, and, if so, what diagnosis was made? Is there a prior history of bipolar illness, depression, schizophrenia, malingering, or conversion disorder? Is there a family psychiatric history? Is there a history of prior severe psychologic trauma, post-traumatic stress disorder, or dissociative states? Mutism may be the presenting sign of any of these psychiatric illnesses.

Have signs of catatonia been witnessed?
Posturing, stereotypy, waxy flexibility, automatic obedience, negativism, extremity rigidity, echolalia, echopraxia, and stupor are all signs of catatonia.

Because true mutism more often occurs with catatonia than without, the absence of catatonic signs should alert the clinician to consider other causes of the communication deficit, such as a metabolic disturbance or aphasia from a cerebral lesion. Note, however, that mutism from conversion disorder, dissociation, and malingering often presents without catatonia.

What medications has the patient taken previously and most recently?
A particular group of patients develop mutism shortly after starting antipsychotics. Other medications previously linked to mutism with catatonia include maprotiline hydrochloride and aspirin in toxic doses. Additionally, corticosteroids have been linked to mutism without catatonia. Severe hypnotic or anxiolytic withdrawal-induced delirium tremens may be mistakenly misdiagnosed as mutism or catatonia.

Use of insulin, oral hypoglycemics, cholesterol-lowering agents, platelet aggregation inhibitors, anticoagulants, cardiac antiarrhythmics, or antihypertensives indicate an underlying disease predisposing to stroke. Use of antiepileptic drugs should raise vigilance for absence seizures or postictal mutism.

Slurred speech is frequently seen in the context of oversedation and ataxia from medication toxicity. This may be caused by any potentially sedating or anticholinergic medication and is more commonly seen in geriatric patients.

Is there a history of drug abuse?

Phencyclidine hydrochloride (PCP)-induced psychosis and alcohol-induced psychosis can produce mutism with catatonia.

In a child, is the mutism selective to certain situations?

Mutism in children is most commonly selective. It generally occurs between the ages of 3 and 8 years as a failure to speak in school or to adults outside the home. The onset is gradual, and these children have typically been excessively shy, inhibited, or anxious previously.

Behavior not characteristic of selective mutism, such as not talking to immediate family members, abrupt cessation of speech in one environment, or absence of speech in all settings, should raise concerns about other causes of mutism. Mutism in a child who never learned to speak is most likely due to a specific or pervasive developmental disorder (e.g., autism) or deafness. Childhood-onset schizophrenia should also be considered. Petit mal seizures in children may closely resemble selective mutism.

Does the patient have risk factors for stroke, including prior stroke, older age, poorly controlled diabetes, hypertension, cigarette smoking, or a family history of stroke?

Aphasias are most often due to embolic infarction of the middle cerebral artery. Aphasias can be divided largely into impaired verbal language output (motor aphasias) and impaired language syntax and comprehension (sensory aphasias).

Has there been a history of recent hypoxia or prolonged hypotension?

Recent hypoxia or prolonged hypotension may result in transcortical motor or sensory aphasias, caused by lesions of the so-called watershed area between the blood supply of the anterior communicating artery and the middle cerebral artery or between the middle and the posterior cerebral arteries.

In cases of incomprehensive disordered language, can other classic signs of psychiatric illness be identified?

On rare occasions, a sensory aphasia may produce disordered

language that needs distinction from a psychotic thought disorder. The sensory aphasias are problems with language reception and comprehension (also called **posterior aphasias**). Both Wernicke's aphasia and transcortical sensory aphasia present with a normal amount of verbal output (unlike motor aphasia) but with syntactical errors such as paraphasias. Because people with sensory aphasia lack language comprehension, they are initially unaware of the deficit and may even become agitated or paranoid as they are blamed for communication difficulties. On occasion, more severely affected patients may present with incomprehensive language full of jargon that is mistakenly attributed to a psychotic thought disorder. These patients will usually lack the poverty of thought, bizarre thinking, delusions, or hallucinations typical of psychotic disorders, making the distinction clear.

Have other neurologic etiologies of mutism been considered?

In **akinetic mutism,** extensive bilateral anterior frontal lobe disease is accompanied by a reduction in all drive to action and psychomotor activity, ranging from abulia in milder forms to akinetic mutism, the most severe form. Although these patients register most of what is happening around them and form memories, they can lie totally motionless and silent for days or weeks at a time. Akinetic mutism has also been associated with third ventricular lesions and unilateral dominant frontal lobe lesions.

Aphemia (or "pure word mutism") is an occasionally seen transient loss of all capacity to speak due to a vascular or other localized lesion of the dominant frontal lobe. Unlike in Broca's aphasia, writing and inner speech (reading silently) remain undisturbed. A facial/brachial paresis may be associated. The most distinctive feature of this aphasia is the resolution of normal language within weeks or months. Often recovery includes a period of dysarthria.

The **"locked in" syndrome** is a rare neurologic state with a complete inability to respond in any way, verbal or nonverbal, yet with no alteration in awareness or consciousness. This syndrome stems most commonly from a lesion of the basis pontis affecting corticobulbar and corticospinal pathways necessary for response but sparing pathways responsible for arousal. Severe degrees of motor neuropathy (e.g., Guillain-Barré syndrome) or periodic paralysis may present similarly.

Is there a history of tertiary syphilis, encephalitis, epilepsy, basal ganglia disorders, or endocrine disorders, including hyperparathyoridism, myxedema, diabetic ketoacidosis, and Addison's disease?

All of these have been reported to have caused mutism.

Assessment of Speech and Communication

Is the patient entirely mute, or can the patient make attempts at verbal communication? Can the patient repeat?

Patients with true psychogenic mutism do not attempt verbal communication. On the contrary, patients with aphasias, no matter how severe, are never entirely silent. Although they may have tremendous difficulty getting words out, patients with aphasia can make some sounds, even if restricted to crude syllabic stereotypies, repeated explicatives, or grunts.

Those with abulia or akinetic mutism have no motivation and thus do not attempt communication spontaneously. They may, however, be able to repeat what the examiner says.

In both pure Broca's motor aphasia and Wernicke's sensory aphasia, patients cannot repeat properly. On the contrary, patients with transcortical motor aphasia may not initiate spontaneous conversational speech beyond a few grunts, yet they can repeat normally. Similarly, patients with transcortical sensory aphasia can repeat normally.

Can the patient write?

Patients with severe Broca's aphasia cannot write. Patient's with aphemia can write. Patients with abulia or akinetic mutism may write (depending on severity of amotivation). Patients with catatonia generally do not write. Patients with mutism as part of a conversion disorder or malingering often can write. Patients with loss of only vocal apparatus (i.e., laryngitis, vocal cord tumor, or paralysis) or muscles of articulation certainly can write.

Can the patient whisper or make lip movements of speech?

The ability to whisper or move the lips may help to identify or eliminate the presence of a bilateral vocal cord paralysis or a severe articulation deficit.

Selective Neurologic Examination

Assessment of every new-onset change in speech or communication should include a neurologic examination. This is particularly critical for older patients and for patients without prior known psychiatric illness, as organic causes of mutism may be overlooked. A neurologic examination can help determine if the change in speech or communication exists as part of catatonia, aphasia, or dysarthria.

General Appearance

On observation, does the patient demonstrate any marked psychomotor abnormalities?

Abnormal posturing or stereotyped movements may point toward catatonia.

Face and Eyes

Is the pupillary diameter abnormal? Are pupils reactive to light?

Abnormal pupillary size or reactivity may be seen in drug intoxication or withdrawal states or in brain stem lesions. A psychiatric cause of mutism should be suspected in patients who resist eye opening.

Are there abnormalities in facial musculature?

Focal central nervous system (CNS) lesions affecting language production may also cause decreased voluntary control of muscles of facial expression or of oral/vocal regions (as the two functions stem from nearby areas in the brain).

Can the patient still whistle or form words with his or her lips?

Check for facial asymmetry or an asymmetric smile.

Is tongue protrusion midline?

Remember, the tongue will deviate to the side of the lesion.

Assessment of phonation, articulation, and nonspeech movements such as swallowing or cough should be assessed to rule out failure of the peripheral sensorimotor speech apparatus.

Extremities

Is there bilateral extremity rigidity?

This may be indicative of catatonia, NMS, or severe extrapyramidal symptoms (EPS) from antipsychotics or from Parkinson's disease, all of which may present with mutism.

Is there waxy flexibility of the limbs, as seen in catatonia?

Is there unilateral weakness, spasticity, or exaggerated reflexes?

Patients with impaired speech from motor aphasia will often demonstrate these signs in the contralateral upper extremity and sometimes in the lower extremity.

Are primitive reflexes elicited?

Degeneration or lesions of the frontal lobes can produce the so-called frontal release signs such as snout, suckling, grasp, or rooting reflexes. Similarly, check for the Babinski reflex.

Diagnostic Tests

Neuroimaging

Acute new-onset language disturbance or dysarthria in the geriatric population often requires immediate neuroimaging to rule out a vascular event. For any suspected acute cerebral hemor-rhage, an immediate noncontrast head computed tomography (CT) scan is indicated. Similarly, for suspected evolving ischemic stroke, a noncontrast head CT scan is generally preferred over magnetic resonance imaging (MRI) for its ease and rapidity; re-member, however, that clinical signs may precede the ability to detect an evolving stroke with CT scanning initially. MRI, al-though more expensive and time-consuming, is a more sensitive tool to confirm suspicion of the vast majority of CNS lesions of all kinds. Cost aside, it is generally preferred in nonemergent cases.

Laboratory Studies

Impaired speech in the context of a fluctuating level of con-sciousness may signify a delirium or drug intoxication and re-quires appropriate laboratory assessment (see Chapter 13).

Electroencephalography

Electroencephalography (EEG) may confirm suspected ongoing epileptic activity or a metabolic encephalopathy causing a change in communication.

Additional Diagnostic Techniques

Lorazepam, parenterally given, will often improve symptoms of catatonia. A typical starting dose is **lorazepam 2 mg intramus-cularly (IM) or 1 mg intravenously (IV)**. This may require up-ward titration of dose. Benzodiazepines will also generally im-prove delirium specifically from alcohol, barbiturate, or benzodiazepine withdrawal or from epileptic activity. Use cau-tion, however, because benzodiazepines will generally worsen most delirium and dementia, and it may worsen depression.

The Amytal Sodium interview may be used to provide diagnos-tically useful information but should also be performed with caution, particularly for suspected delirium or dementia. Cata-tonic patients may have lucid response periods. Patients with hysteria may reveal the cause of their distress.

■ MANAGEMENT

- **Suspected delirium:** Proper laboratory and neuroimaging as-sessment are essential. Medical consultation and management may be necessary, particularly in cases of impaired vital signs.
- **Suspected evolving stroke:** An immediate noncontrast head CT scan and neurologic consultation are necessary.
- **Depression:** Mutism may stem from severe psychomotor re-tardation. The patient may lack the energy to express thoughts or may have markedly slowed thinking. Mute pa-tients may also be psychotically depressed. Psychotic depres-

sion generally requires an antipsychotic and an antidepressant.

- **Schizophrenia:** Patients with schizophrenia show poverty of thought, energy, or motivation. They may be too frightened to speak, may be completely preoccupied by internal stimuli, or may have bizarre beliefs that entail silence. They may be paralyzed by ambivalence. Treatment with an antipsychotic should resolve mutism over time.
- **Recent antipsychotic exposure:** For severe parkinsonism, consider giving an anticholinergic such as **benztropine 2 mg PO or IM** or **diphenhydramine 50 mg PO or IM.** Also rule out NMS; patients with NMS present with extreme rigidity, altered level of consciousness, autonomic instability, fever, and elevated creatinine kinase level.
- **Mutism in acute drug psychosis:** Manage mutism in acute drug psychosis with a benzodiazepine such as **lorazepam 1 to 2 mg PO or IM every 4 to 6 hours as needed.** Antipsychotics may be used adjunctively in cases of severe agitation.
- **Selective mutism:** A common treatment approach to selective mutism is behavior modification. General supportive counseling, psychotherapy, speech therapy, and psychopharmacology have all been used as interventions.

General Guidelines for Dealing With Mutism of a Psychiatric Etiology

- Frequent brief contacts may be more useful than long interviews.
- Simple, concrete questions evoke better responses than do complex, open-ended questions.
- Surreptitious observation is important.
- Nursing and social work staff who spend extensive time with the patient and show empathic concern may gain information more readily.
- One-to-one observation may be necessary if dangerousness cannot be assessed.

Additional Considerations in Catatonia

Patients with catatonia may require nutritional support. Intravenous fluid replacement may be indicated initially, and ongoing monitoring of oral food intake, fluid intake and output, weight, and electrolytes may be needed. Some patients with catatonia may require treatment of self-inflicted injuries.

Unresponsive catatonic patients are awake and alert and should have actions explained to them. Patients in a catatonic stupor may suddenly and without warning became extremely excited, agitated, and potentially violent. In dangerous cases, emergency treatment will generally include IM injection of an antipsychotic such as **haloperidol (Haldol) 2 to 5 mg** or **fluphenazine 2 to 5 mg. Lorazepam 1 to 2 mg IM** may be combined with the antipsychotic for additional sedation as necessary. In addition to IV/IM lorazepam, electroconvulsive therapy is often an effective treatment for catatonia.

16 | Physical and Sexual Trauma

VAN YU

Victims of trauma often require urgent psychiatric and medical attention. Here, **trauma** is an event or events that would fulfill the *Diagnostic and Statistical Manual of Mental Disorders*, 4th edition (DSM-IV), criterion A for post-traumatic stress disorder or acute stress disorder: "an event or events that involved actual or threatened death or serious injury, or a threat to the physical integrity of self or others."* This chapter is a brief guide for the psychiatric consultant on how to provide psychiatric intervention in the hours after acute trauma. This intervention aims to reduce the morbidity associated with post-traumatic stress disorder and acute stress disorder. As in the first edition of this book, a consideration of the acute management of the female victim of rape is used to illustrate basic principles that can be applied to crisis intervention in general. Brief comments about special considerations for other populations will follow.

■ RAPE OF WOMEN

In 1995, 72 of every 100,000 women in the United States were reported to be a victim of rape. Because of underreporting, however, this number probably represents only about half of the true incidence of rape. As with the vast majority of trauma victims, acute medical attention is the first priority for the victim of rape. Therefore, the physician should be familiar with all medical interventions expected of the psychiatric consultant.

■ PHONE CALL

Questions

1. What is the behavior of the patient?

A review of the criteria for post-traumatic stress disorder and acute stress disorder should convince the psychiatric consultant that there could be a wide range of behavior after trauma. Of immediate concern, however, is agitated

---

*See "Diagnostic criteria for 309.81 Posttraumatic Stress Disorder" and "Diagnostic criteria for 308.3 Acute Stress Disorder" in DSM-IV.

behavior that may require intervention before the psychiatric consultant can arrive.

2. Does the patient have any injuries?

Although psychiatric intervention for rape is important, rape is a violent act that also requires immediate medical evaluation.

3. What are the patient's vital signs?

Again, rape is violent, and medical evaluation is the first priority. Also, there is a significant association between alcohol and substance use, violence, and accidents. Abnormal vital signs may be a first clue that alcohol or substance use is involved.

Orders

1. Ask for the patient's old chart. Even though rape is the chief complaint, this patient like any other may have other significant medical or psychiatric conditions.
2. In addition to a rape victim's primary treatment team, most hospitals have a crime or rape victim team that should be summoned as soon as possible. Also ask to see any law enforcement officials involved with the case.
3. One-to-one observation is prudent until you can evaluate the patient.
4. Agitated patients may require intervention before the psychiatric consultant is able to arrive, especially if a patient's agitation poses an acute danger to self or others. One dose of a benzodiazepine, for example, **lorazepam 1 to 2 mg** or **diazepam 5 to 10 mg orally or parenterally,** may be given.

Inform RN

"Will arrive in . . . minutes."

■ ELEVATOR THOUGHTS

The two major psychiatric diagnoses to consider for victims of trauma are post-traumatic stress disorder and acute stress disorder. A brief review of the criteria for these disorders should convince the physician that he or she might expect a variety of symptoms, including dissociative phenomena. Although post-traumatic stress disorder will not be a diagnosis this early in the presentation, psychiatric intervention is aimed at reducing the morbidity that can occur later from this condition.

The trauma or rape victim may also meet criteria for adjustment disorder or major depressive disorder some time after the trauma.

■ MAJOR THREAT TO LIFE

As mentioned earlier, a medical evaluation is the first priority. As the psychiatric consultant, you are obliged to pay particular attention to the patient's level of consciousness and orientation as these might indicate medical or neurologic problems. Consider the possible role of alcohol or substance use contributing to a patient's mental status.

Suicidality and homicidality are especially significant concerns because the patient's judgment may be impaired by the psychologic shock of the trauma and/or by alcohol or substance intoxication.

■ BEDSIDE

Quick Look Test

It is imperative to assess the patient's level of consciousness and orientation.

Airway and Vital Signs

Abnormal vital signs can be a clue to an inapparent medical or neurologic injury or to alcohol or substance intoxication or withdrawal.

Selective History

During any stage in the evaluation and treatment of a rape or trauma victim, it is important to help the patient feel as free as possible to discuss details of the rape and her reactions to it. Pay special attention to avoid statements that the patient may experience as judgmental. Also, it is not the psychiatric consultant's job to determine the accuracy of the patient's story; eliciting the patient's experience of the trauma is much more important.

Part of the trauma of rape is the experience of helplessness during the attack. You can start to restore a patient's feeling of empowerment and physical integrity simply by asking permission to interview her.

A rape victim will be involved in a criminal investigation. In addition to speaking with the psychiatric consultant and other members of a primary treatment team, a rape victim will also experience the potentially traumatic experience of speaking with a rape or crime victim team and with law enforcement officials. Being able to provide your patient with detailed information about the criminal investigation she faces, including informing her of her right to press charges, can ease some anxiety about what might otherwise be a bewildering process. Remember that anything you document is potential evidence in the criminal investigation.

Rape and trauma victims can experience a wide variety of psychiatric symptoms, including dissociative symptoms and psychosis. Alcohol and substance intoxication might also contribute to the patient's mental status. Suicidal or homicidal ideation may be present and can be especially worrisome if neurologic injury, intoxication, or other acute psychiatric symptoms impair the victim's judgment. Patients may also express psychiatric symptoms in the form of somatic complaints.

Because your acute management of the rape or trauma victim include the patient's social supports, take careful note of available family and friends.

Selective Physical Examination

The psychiatric consultant will likely not be directly involved in the physical examination. The physical examination of a rape victim not only serves the traditional purpose of evaluating the need for medical intervention but also is a primary source of physical evidence for the criminal investigation. Most hospitals have a "rape kit" for this purpose. The physical examination can itself be traumatic. Remove as many people from the examination room as possible, and whenever possible, have a woman examine a female patient (at the very least a woman should be present). Remember that photograph taking may be a part of the physical examination.

■ MANAGEMENT

Some patients may be too agitated to cooperate with a psychiatric evaluation. If a patient's agitation represents an acute danger to self or others, acute pharmacologic intervention may be necessary. The benzodiazepine **lorazepam 1 to 2 mg parenterally or orally** or **diazepam 5 to 10 mg parenterally or orally** is safe for almost all patients.

For the patient who can participate in a psychiatric interview, acute intervention is aimed at reducing the morbidity associated with acute stress disorder and post-traumatic stress disorder. (A significant number of victims of rape are found later to meet the criteria for post-traumatic stress disorder.)

Traumatic stress leads to the development of coping mechanisms, including affective numbing and dissociation, that may become debilitating later. Cognitive-behavioral techniques are designed to help the patient process trauma before these maladaptive coping mechanisms can form and become entrenched.

The psychiatric consultant can lay the groundwork for cognitive processing therapy in the hours after rape or other trauma. Supportive interventions as basic as consoling and comforting help the patient feel safe and help prevent generalization of fear and anxiety to the surrounding environment. Education about post-traumatic stress disorder demystifies the experiencing of unfamiliar psychiatric sequelae of trauma and provides cognitive building blocks for the patient to begin to be able to gain control over these symptoms. Providing a nonjudgmental forum to speak about the trauma sets the stage for cognitive processing that the patient will be encouraged to do in cognitive-behavioral therapy.

Most patients will benefit from some type of ongoing therapy after rape or other trauma. Therefore, it is imperative as part of acute psychiatric intervention to provide a plan for the patient to seek follow-up treatment.

Finally, the psychiatric consultant must judge how safe it is for the rape or trauma victim to leave the hospital. This judgment is based on the relative significance of psychiatric symptoms, including suicidality and homicidality, alcohol or substance intoxication, medical or neurologic injury, and the availability of social supports including family and friends.

■ SPECIAL CONSIDERATIONS FOR OTHER POPULATIONS

Child Abuse

For the child presenting to the emergency department after trauma, child abuse will rarely be the presenting complaint. Often the possibility of child abuse is entertained only after the pediatrician providing medical care discovers physical injuries that are not consistent with the presenting complaint and history provided by the parents or other adults. One common physical clue is a bathing-suit pattern of bruises, so-called because of a distribution that is not apparent to a casual observer (see Appendix L).

Depending on the age of the child, obtaining a verbal history may be difficult. Also, the child may resist providing information because of fear of retribution by the abuser. The use of dolls or drawing during the psychiatric interview is helpful.

It is also important to interview a child's parents, siblings, or other caretakers. Keep in mind that abusers will likely not provide accurate information. Also remember when interviewing adult caretakers that there is a significant association between psychiatric illness or substance use and child abuse.

Child abuse will not always be the result of violence or neglect. Some parents or caretakers cause medical illnesses in children (i.e., Munchausen's syndrome by proxy).

All states have laws concerning the mandated reporting of child abuse that the psychiatric consultant should be familiar with. Also, most hospitals have a child abuse team that should be contacted if there is a suspicion of child abuse.

Spouse Abuse

As with children, victims of spouse abuse will often not present to the emergency department with this complaint. Again, suspicious physical injuries including a bathing-suit pattern of bruises will be clues.

The vast majority of victims of spouse abuse are women. Also, for any given couple, the risk of spouse abuse increases during pregnancy.

Elder Abuse

The evaluation of elder abuse is very similar to the evaluation of child abuse (see Appendix M). Often the victim of elder abuse will not be able to provide history because of a medical or neurologic illness, necessitating the interview of caretakers.

Many states have laws about the mandated reporting of elder abuse that the psychiatric consultant should be familiar with.

Survivors of Disasters

For survivors of disasters, feeling helpless in the face of calamity is an especially significant experience. You can help start the process of restoring a sense of control to survivors by attending to concrete issues such as physical safety, food, and shelter, and using supportive interventions such as consoling and comforting. Disaster survivors often experience survivor guilt based on the randomness of who has survived. The root of survivor guilt is a cognitive distortion that the psychiatric consultant can target by challenging the feelings of responsibility that many survivors have. Delivering psychiatric intervention to a group of survivors is often beneficial as members of the group can provide support for each other and help the psychiatric consultant challenge cognitive distortions.

Rescue Workers, Law Enforcement Officials, and Other Emergency Service Workers

Emergency service workers are often reluctant to seek psychiatric consultation after a traumatic event. To circumvent reluctance, team leaders often employ "critical incident stress debriefing" (CISD) as a formalized, mandatory way to deliver psychiatric intervention. A review of the steps of CISD (Table 16–1) should

Table 16–1 □ **PHASES OF CRITICAL INCIDENT STRESS DEBRIEFING (CISD)**

Introduction
Clinician describes frame of debriefing, including limits of confidentiality and proposed benefits

Facts
Group members describe their roles and tasks during the incident and describe what happened

Thoughts
Group members express their first thoughts during the incident, with the aim of eliciting a more personal perspective

Reactions
Group members express the worst part of the experience. This aims to encourage people to acknowledge and express their reactions and feelings

Symptoms
Group members review their own symptoms or cognitive, physical, emotional, and behavioral distress

Teaching
Clinician emphasizes normality of symptoms and gives information about symptom management

Relating
Clinician wraps up meeting

Adapted from Raphael B, Wilson J, Meldrum L, McFarlane AC: Acute preventive interventions. In Van der Kolk BA, McFarlane AC, Weisaeth L (eds): Traumatic Stress. New York, The Guilford Press, 1996, p 468.

convince the clinician that CISD comes from the same theoretical framework and has the same goals as the cognitive-behavioral techniques described earlier. In the emergency department, the psychiatric consultant may find workers less reluctant to participate in group sessions rather than individual counseling sessions.

Bibliography

Calhoun KS, Resick PA: Post-traumatic stress disorder. In Barlow DH (ed): Clinical Handbook of Psychological Disorders, 2nd ed. New York, The Guilford Press, 1993, pp 48–98.

Kaplan HI, Sadock BJ (eds): Pocket Handbook of Emergency Psychiatric Medicine. Baltimore, Williams & Wilkins, 1993.

Van der Kolk BA, McFarlane AC, Weisaeth L (eds): Traumatic Stress. New York, The Guilford Press, 1996.

Welsh CJ: Crisis intervention. In Bernstein CA, Ladds BJ, Maloney AS, Weiner ED (eds): On Call Psychiatry. Philadelphia, WB Saunders Co, 1997, pp 83–92.

SCOTT BIENENFELD
M. BREALYN SELLERS

Substance abuse is a major part of any thorough psychiatric evaluation. Our understanding of the neurobiologic mechanisms of addiction progressed rapidly in the 1990s. Although we now have a more complex understanding of the intricacies of abuse and dependence, an intoxicated patient remains one of the most difficult psychiatric challenges to the psychiatrist on call. Often, intoxicated patients are behaviorally difficult and may present with potentially life-threatening conditions; hence they require immediate attention. Although these patients may appear to have a primary psychiatric disorder, intoxication must clear before other diagnoses can be considered.*

This chapter will guide you in identifying and managing intoxication syndromes. Obtaining a thorough history is key to providing care quickly and effectively.

■ PHONE CALL

Questions

1. What is the level of consciousness?
2. What are the vital signs?
3. What were the substances used?
4. How much was used?
5. How long ago was the last use?
6. What is the behavior?

Orders

Measure blood alcohol level and obtain urine toxicology results immediately.

Inform RN

"Will arrive in . . . minutes."

---

*See "Criteria for Substance Intoxication" in the *Diagnostic and Statistical Manual of Mental Disorders,* 4th edition (DSM-IV).

■ ELEVATOR THOUGHTS

What substances has the person been using?

You should first consider the category of drug ingested. These most commonly include alcohol, hallucinogens, inhalants, marijuana, opiates, psychostimulants, and sedative-hypnotics. Often more than one substance will be involved. Street drugs have the added complication of not being pure, often containing additives and mixtures of drugs. Be aware of a mixed withdrawal and intoxication state. In general, intoxicated patients can be divided into two categories: lethargic or obtunded patients and agitated or restless patients.

If the patient appears lethargic or is in a coma, suspect intoxication from

1. Opiates: meperidine (Demerol), morphine, heroin, opium, methadone, pentazocine (Talwin)
2. Sedative-hypnotics: barbiturates, benzodiazepines, nonbarbiturate sedatives, glutethimide (Doriden), meprobamate (Equanil, Miltown)
3. Alcohol

If the patient is described as restless or agitated, suspect intoxication from

1. Alcohol
2. Psychostimulants: cocaine, amphetamine
3. Hallucinogens: phencyclidine hydrochloride (PCP), lysergic acid diethylamide (LSD), marijuana, methylenedioxymethamphetamine (MDMA, "Ecstasy")
4. Over-the-counter agents and natural remedies: diphenhydramine, ma-huang, kava kava, valerian root, and so forth

■ BEDSIDE

Quick Look Test

What is the patient's appearance and level of activity?

What is the patient's level of consciousness?

What is the patient's history (enlist friends and relatives if necessary)?

Vital Signs

What are the patient's vital signs?

Selective History

1. What substances were inhaled, ingested, or injected?
2. How much was used?

3. How long ago was the last use?
4. Does the patient habitually use the substance? If so, how much and how often? It is characteristic of chronic substance abusers to underreport the extent of their use.
5. Does the patient use over-the-counter remedies?

Selective Physical Examination

1. Pupils
2. Tremors
3. Mental status examination
4. Neurologic examination

Substance-Specific Intoxication Syndromes

Alcohol

Signs and symptoms include the following:
1. Slurred speech
2. Ataxia
3. Disinhibition
4. Aggression
5. Tachycardia
6. Hypothermia
7. Nystagmus
8. Coma

General management involves the following:
1. Evaluate the patient in a quiet area.
2. Monitor vital signs.
3. Be aware of potential agitation and violence. Treat such behavior with benzodiazepines, such as **lorazepam 1 to 2 mg orally (PO) or intramuscularly (IM) every 4 hours.**
4. Patients whom you suspect of using excessive alcohol should be given **thiamine (100 mg IM then PO for 6 days)** to prevent the onset of Wernicke's encephalopathy. **Folate 1 mg PO should be given for 7 days.** Patients with other vitamin B deficiencies should be given supplements appropriately.
5. Treat unconscious patients supportively, starting with intravenous (IV) fluids and glucose; maintain airway, and monitor vital signs.

Serious Alcohol Intoxication

A person with a blood alcohol level of 0.1 to 0.15 mg/dL is considered legally intoxicated. A level of 0.3 to 0.4 mg/dL will cause coma and other problems.

Management involves the following:
1. Gastric lavage
2. **Thiamine 100 mg IM** for prophylaxis against Wernicke's encephalopathy
3. Fifty milliliters of 50% glucose to prevent hypoglycemia
4. Intensive care unit (ICU) monitoring
5. Monitoring for withdrawal symptoms (see Chapter 18)

Psychostimulants (Cocaine, Amphetamines)

Signs and symptoms include the following:
1. Restlessness
2. Euphoria
3. Psychosis, hallucinations
4. Decreased appetite
5. Hypertension
6. Dilated, reactive pupils
7. Cardiac arrhythmias, tachycardia
8. Fever
9. Seizures
10. Coma

Chronic high-dose cocaine users may exhibit paranoia that can mimic schizophrenia. A patient who has used extremely high doses may exhibit autonomic instability and hyperthermia, which may progress to seizures, strokes, and death.

General management involves the following:
1. Evaluate in a quiet area.
2. Mild symptoms should be managed by reassuring the patient.
3. Benzodiazepines can be used for acute agitation. Use **lorazepam (Ativan) 1 to 2 mg as often as every 1 to 2 hours (generally not to exceed 8 mg in a 24-hour period)** until the patient has calmed down.
4. Severely paranoid or agitated patients should also receive antipsychotic medications, such as **haloperidol (Haldol) 5 mg every 30 minutes until the patient has calmed down (up to ~20 mg in a 14-hour period).**
5. Be aware of medical complications, such as myocardial infarction, stroke, and intracranial hemorrhage.
6. Severe adrenergic reactions (diaphoresis, tachycardia, hyperpyrexia, hypertension) should be treated with beta-blockers, such as **propranolol (Inderal) 20 to 40 mg PO or 1 to 2 mg IV,** except in patients with asthma, diabetes, or cardiovascular disease.
7. Any temperature greater than 102°F is a medical emergency and should be treated aggressively with a cooling blanket and other measures.

8. Seizures should be treated as any other seizure with **IV diazepam (Valium) 5 to 20 mg per minute and repeated at 15-minute intervals as necessary.**
9. If the paranoid behavior persists for longer than 12 hours, hospitalization should be considered. Otherwise, discharge to a responsible person may be appropriate. An immediate follow-up appointment may be considered.
10. Acidifying the urine with ascorbic acid (vitamin C) or ammonium chloride will increase excretion.

Caffeine

Signs and symptoms mimic those caused by stimulants. Manage the patient symptomatically.

Marijuana (Cannabis)

Signs and symptoms include the following:
1. Euphoria, silliness, feeling of well-being
2. Altered perceptions
3. Lack of coordination
4. Increased appetite, thirst
5. Tachycardia
6. Injected conjunctivae
7. Increased anxiety, paranoia

Management involves the following:
1. Reassure the patient that the effects will subside.
2. Treat acute anxiety with benzodiazepines such as **lorazepam 1 to 2 mg PO every 1 to 2 hours as needed (do not exceed 8 mg in a 24-hour period).**

Hallucinogens

Hallucinogens include LSD, psilocybin (mushrooms), dimethoxymethylamphetamine (STP or DOM), mescaline (peyote), diethyltryptamine (DET), dimethyltryptamine (DMT), and methylenedioxymethamphetamine ("Ecstasy").

Signs and symptoms include the following:
1. Extreme, labile effect
2. Cyclic reactions with alternating periods of lucidity and hallucinations
3. Perceptual distortions, including hallucinations, and synesthesia, in which, for example, sound is perceived as color
4. Dilated pupils
5. Tachycardia, palpitations
6. Diaphoresis
7. Tremor, incoordination
8. Hypertension
9. Hyperthermia
10. Piloerection

The effects mostly occur over 6 to 12 hours but may last up to several days. One common emergency room presentation is that of a patient having a "bad trip," which is an adverse drug reaction following the use of hallucinogenic drugs. Manifestations may vary from an acute panic reaction to a temporary psychotic state. The patient may report feelings of helplessness, fear of losing control, fear of going crazy, and suspiciousness that can reach proportions of frank paranoia. Patients may also complain of intense anxiety, depression, and hallucinations, predominantly visual.

Flashbacks are another unique presentation that may occur with chronic LSD use. A flashback is a spontaneous recurrence of the original LSD trip. It usually occurs suddenly and lasts from several minutes to several hours.

Management involves the following:

1. Reassurance is the most important therapeutic intervention.
2. Do not leave the patient alone because behavior can become dangerous.
3. Treat with **lorazepam 1 to 2 mg PO or IM every 1 to 2 hours until the patient has calmed down.**
4. Consider hospitalization when the reaction lasts longer than 24 hours despite vigorous intervention.
5. Discharge into the custody of friends or family with appropriate follow-up.

"Ecstasy"

Methylenedioxymethamphetamine (MDMA, "E," "X") has become a very popular drug among young adults and adolescents, particularly in the "club/rave scene." In the emergency setting, clinicians often forget to ask about "club drugs." While the risk of death from MDMA remains low, MDMA overdose can lead to hyperthermia and dehydration, especially when users have been awake for long periods of time with decreased fluid intake (e.g., dancing for extended periods in hot, enclosed places). In rare cases, MDMA overdose can produce a syndrome similar to neuroleptic malignant syndrome (NMS), characterized by rigidity, hyperthermia, dehydration, mental status changes, rhabdomyolysis leading to renal failure, convulsions, and autonomic dysregulation. There have been reports of disseminated intravascular coagulation (DIC) resulting from extreme hyperthermia related to MDMA overdose.

If MDMA overdose is suspected, the condition should be treated promptly. Management involves the following:

1. Rehydration is imperative to prevent renal failure.
2. Electrolytes should be monitored closely.
3. Hyperthermia should be corrected (cooling blankets).
4. Ask for a medical consultation.

Inhalants

Signs and symptoms include the following:
1. Altered states of consciousness ranging from euphoria to clouding of consciousness
2. Dizziness, syncope
3. Psychosis
4. Nausea, vomiting, epigastric distress
5. Chest pain
6. Tachycardia, ventricular fibrillation
7. Organ damage (brain, liver, kidney, heart)
8. Odor on the breath

Acute intoxication can last from 15 to 45 minutes. Drowsiness and stupor may last for hours.

Management involves the following:
1. Attempt to identify the solvent. Leaded gasoline may require the use of a chelating agent.
2. Restoration of oxygenation should resolve symptoms within minutes.
3. Treat acute psychosis with **haloperidol 2 to 5 mg PO or IM.**

Opioids

Opioids include opium, morphine, heroin, meperidine, methadone, pentazocine, and propoxyphene (Darvon). Signs and symptoms include the following:
1. Pinpoint pupils unresponsive to light, except with meperidine, which may produce dilated pupils
2. Depressed respiration and level of consciousness
3. Bradycardia
4. Hypothermia
5. Pulmonary edema

Overdose is a medical emergency because of pulmonary edema and respiratory depression and requires treatment in the intensive care unit.

Management involves the following:
1. Support the airway.
2. Treat with **naloxone 0.4 to 2.0 mg IV every 2 to 3 minutes until respirations are stable.** After **10 mg,** consider other causes for symptomatology.
3. The half-life of naloxone is much shorter than that of most opioids (approximately 1 hour), so observe closely for the re-emergence of symptoms (e.g., coma) and re-treat with naloxone; failure to do so may result in patient death after release from the emergency room.
4. Monitor for withdrawal symptoms (see Chapter 18).

Phencyclidine

Signs and symptoms include the following:
1. Nystagmus, ataxia, dysarthria

2. Hyperreflexia, numbness
3. Disorientation, memory impairment
4. Hallucinations, synesthesia
5. Decreased sensitivity to pain
6. Rigidity
7. Hypertension
8. Tachycardia
9. Stupor
10. Seizures
11. Coma, death

Management involves the following:
1. Consider hospitalization; overdose can be fatal.
2. Minimize sensory stimulation. Attempts to reassure the patient may aggravate the situation.
3. Treat psychosis with **haloperidol 2 to 5 mg PO or IM every hour until the patient is calm.**
4. Treat anxiety or agitation with **lorazepam 1 to 2 mg PO or IM every 30 to 60 minutes until the patient is calm.**
5. Acidify urine with ascorbic acid or ammonium chloride.
6. Monitor closely because large ingestions may result in coma and death.
7. Vital signs and pulmonary and cardiovascular functioning must be observed and supported when necessary.

Sedative-Hypnotics

Sedative-hypnotics include barbiturates (phenobarbital, secobarbital), nonbarbiturates, glutethimide, and meprobamate.

Signs and symptoms include the following:
1. Ataxia
2. Slurred speech
3. Nystagmus
4. Confusion
5. Decreased respiration
6. Decreased level of consciousness
7. Hypotension

Be aware of overdose with glutethimide. Patients need to be observed closely after emergence from a coma because the drug is stored in the fat tissues. As more drug is released by the tissue stores, patients may lapse back into coma.

Management involves the following:
1. Consider hospitalization; overdose can be fatal. Sluggishness or coma represents a life-threatening emergency.
2. Monitor vital signs and support the airway as needed.
3. If the patient is awake, keep awake.
4. There is no specific antidote, but use gastric lavage if the drug was taken in the last 4 to 6 hours to reduce further absorption.

5. Forced diuresis and dialysis should be considered.
6. Monitor for withdrawal symptoms (see Chapter 18).

Anxiolytics and Benzodiazepines

Signs and symptoms include the following:
1. Confusion
2. Ataxia
3. Slurred speech

Benzodiazepine overdose alone is rarely fatal. Mixture with other drugs, however, particularly alcohol, can cause fatal respiratory depression.

Management involves the following:
1. Monitor vital signs and support the airway as needed.
2. Flumazenil (Romazicon) is a benzodiazepine antagonist that may be used to reverse the effects of an overdose. Secure the airway. Administer **flumazenil 0.2 mg IV through a large vein to minimize pain at the injection site over 30 seconds and then wait 30 seconds. Repeat 0.2 to 0.5 mg over 30 seconds at 1-minute intervals until the patient responds. Do not exceed 3 mg.** Use caution if the patient has taken a concomitant tricyclic antidepressant overdose or if the patient is benzodiazepine dependent because flumazenil may precipitate seizures.

Belladonna Alkaloids

Signs and symptoms are related to the anticholinergic effects (e.g., "red as a beet, dry as a bone, mad as a hatter"):
1. Hot, flushed skin
2. Dry mouth, thirst
3. Blurred vision
4. Confusion, delirium
5. Dilated pupils
6. Tachycardia, arrhythmias
7. Hypertension
8. Urinary retention

Management involves the following:
1. Provide supportive medical management.
2. Discontinue the offending agent.
3. Reassure the patient.
4. Treat agitation with **lorazepam 1 to 2 mg PO or IM every hour until the patient is calm.**
5. For severe medical symptoms or uncontrolled agitation, **physostigmine (Antilirium) 0.5 to 2 mg IM or IV at a slow controlled rate of no more than 1 mg per minute and repeated at intervals of 10 to 30 minutes** can be used to reverse the anticholinergic effects. Use with caution in patients with concomitant medical illness.

Selective Serotonin Reuptake Inhibitors

Signs and symptoms of the serotonin syndrome include the following:

1. Mental status changes (e.g., delirium, anxiety, irritability, confusion)
2. Gastrointestinal disturbance
3. Neurologic changes (e.g., ataxia, tremor, myoclonus, hyperflexia, rigidity)
4. Autonomic nervous system alterations (e.g., hypotension, hypertension, tachycardia, diaphoresis, sialorrhea, mydriasis, tachypnea)
5. Hyperthermia

The syndrome is self-limited and often resolves after discontinuation of the offending agent. In severe cases, supportive measures may be necessary.

Serotonin syndrome and NMS may present with some similar features. A careful history of current medications is therefore essential.

18 | Substance Withdrawal

M. BREALYN SELLERS
SCOTT BIENENFELD

Substance withdrawal is commonly encountered in emergency medicine. The psychiatrist on call is asked to evaluate and treat patients who are behaviorally difficult, suffer clinical stigmata of withdrawal, and complain of various subjective discomforts related to the substance(s) from which they are withdrawing. Emergency stabilization of the patient is the first priority. To diagnose the specific substance withdrawal syndrome, identification of the time course of the symptomatology is imperative. A thorough history and reliable details regarding onset, progression, and relationship to last intake of the substance will help greatly in forming the proper treatment plan. Although many symptoms (e.g., distress, irritability, cognitive impairment, dysphoria) are mild and self-limited, others may progress to life-threatening situations, such as delirium tremens (DTs) and hyperthermia.*

■ PHONE CALL

Questions

1. What are the patient's vital signs?
2. What is the patient's level of consciousness (comatose, obtunded but responsive, disoriented with clouded sensorium, confused, agitated)?
3. Does the patient appear to be in obvious distress? Are objective signs of withdrawal present (piloerection, lacrimation, vomiting, diarrhea, dilated pupils)?
4. Is the patient dangerous to himself or herself or to others, suicidal, or violent?
5. Is there a history of drug use? Are there signs of drug use (e.g., alcohol on breath, needle tracks, vomiting, diarrhea)?
6. If the patient admits to drug use or abuse, what substances were used, when was the last use, how much was used, and by what route was it administered?
7. What medications is the patient using?

---

*See "Criteria for Substance Withdrawal" in the *Diagnostic and Statistical Manual of Mental Disorders,* 4th edition (DSM-IV).

Orders

If the patient is severely agitated, violent, or suicidal, one-to-one observation should be started immediately.

Inform RN

"Will arrive in . . . minutes."
1. If any of the above information is lacking (e.g., vital signs), ask the nurse to obtain it while you are on your way.
2. If indicated, ask the nurse to prepare **lorazepam (Ativan) 2 mg for intramuscular (IM) administration.**

■ ELEVATOR THOUGHTS

What causes substance withdrawal?
Withdrawal from alcohol and sedatives, hypnotics, or anxiolytics, such as barbiturates or benzodiazepines, can be life threatening, whereas withdrawal from opiates is mainly uncomfortable. Consider the possibility of a combination of drugs, especially alcohol in combination with other sedatives or cocaine. Intravenous drug abusers are prone to suffer from other medical complications of their habit. Be alert to possible signs and effects of endocarditis, trauma, intoxication with other substances, and malnutrition. The possibility of infection with the human immunodeficiency virus (HIV) and hepatitis C virus should also be entertained while evaluating and caring for the patient. It is also important to consider feigning of symptoms for secondary gain (to obtain medication, avoid legal consequences, or facilitate hospital admission).

Substance-Specific Syndromes

1. Alcohol withdrawal, including withdrawal delirium (DTs)
2. Sedative, hypnotic, or anxiolytic withdrawal
3. Opioid withdrawal
4. Central nervous system (CNS) stimulant (cocaine and amphetamine) withdrawal
5. Nicotine withdrawal
6. Antidepressant withdrawal
7. Anticholinergic withdrawal

■ MAJOR THREAT TO LIFE

- Withdrawal delirium (DTs)
- CNS depression

- Trauma associated with altered states
- Septic shock, especially in intravenous drug abusers

■ BEDSIDE

Quick Look Test

How does the patient appear?

Is the patient distressed, agitated, somnolent, or comatose? Are there stigmata characteristic of patients who abuse substances?

What is your quick take on the patient's mental status?

Pay special attention to the presence of perceptual disturbances, psychomotor abnormalities, suicidal ideation, violence potential, and affective lability. Include a basic cognitive assessment.

Airway and Vital Signs

Watch for changes in heart rate, blood pressure, respiratory rate, and body temperature.

Selective History and Chart Review

1. Is there a history of recent substance abuse? Has the patient ever had DTs, seizures, shakes, or blackouts?
2. Has the patient been enrolled in detoxification or rehabilitation programs or methadone clinics?

    If the patient is enrolled in a methadone maintenance program, contact the program and obtain the daily maintenance dosage.
3. Is there a psychiatric history of a mood disorder? Has the patient been hospitalized or taken psychotropic medications? Has the patient followed up with treatment?
4. Is the patient a veteran? Has the patient participated in combat? If so, was there substance use while in the military?
5. Is there a family history of substance abuse (e.g., alcoholism in parents)?
6. Is the patient in pain?

    Ask about the localization and quality of pain. Has the patient been prescribed pain medication (e.g., opiates), and for what duration?
7. Is there a history of suicide attempts or violence?

Selective Physical Examination

1. General: Look for piloerection, muscle twitching, and incontinence (postseizure).

2. Neurologic: Check pupil size, sixth cranial nerve palsy, reflexes, psychomotor agitation, and gait.

■ MANAGEMENT: GENERAL

The patient needs a careful medical evaluation to rule out a possible life-threatening situation. This evaluation should include a complete blood count (CBC) and blood chemistry (including liver function tests and thyroid function tests), rapid plasma reagin (RPR), vitamin B_{12}, folate, hepatitis panel, chest x-ray, electrocardiogram (ECG), and head computed tomography (CT) scan (if indicated, to rule out subdural hematoma).

Rule out polysubstance abuse by obtaining urine toxicology and blood alcohol levels, if they have not already been obtained. Some emergency rooms are equipped with dipstick urine toxicology kits.

■ SPECIFIC WITHDRAWAL CONDITIONS

Alcohol Withdrawal

Signs and Symptoms

1. Agitation
2. Hyperactivity
3. Anxiety
4. Hand tremors
5. Nausea or vomiting
6. Insomnia
7. Hallucinations or illusions with clear sensorium
8. Tonic-clonic seizures
9. Increased startle response
10. Increased deep tendon reflexes
11. Orthostatic hypotension

Time Course.   Withdrawal symptoms usually begin when blood concentrations of alcohol decline sharply within 4 to 12 hours after alcohol use has been stopped or reduced. They are related to a hyperadrenergic state. Symptoms peak in intensity during the second day of abstinence and are likely to improve markedly by the fourth or fifth day. Withdrawal is more severe in African Americans, the elderly, and malnourished patients, as well as in those patients with concurrent medical illness.

Immediate Steps

1. Ensure hydration. Encourage fluid intake by mouth (PO) unless disturbances in consciousness are present. Presence

of nausea, vomiting, or diarrhea may prevent effective absorption; in such cases, consider intravenous (IV) fluids.

2. Consider medication. For uncomplicated withdrawal, prescribe a tapered dosage of chlordiazepoxide (Librium) as follows:

Chlordiazepoxide 50 mg PO every 6 hours × 4 doses
Chlordiazepoxide 25 mg PO every 6 hours × 4 doses
Chlordiazepoxide 10 mg PO every 6 hours × 4 doses
Chlordiazepoxide 10 mg PO every 12 hours × 2 doses
Then stop.

Use **chlordiazepoxide 25 mg or 50 mg PO every 6 hours as needed** (PRN) for breakthrough symptoms of withdrawal. Alternatively, **lorazepam 1 mg PO every 2 to 4 hours may be used for the first 24 hours, with an additional 1 mg PO every 2 hours PRN and then slowly tapered over the next week.**

3. Evaluate fluid balance and electrolytes. Correct deficiencies, including calcium, potassium, and magnesium. Intravenous fluids may be necessary.

4. Monitor vital signs and level of consciousness, and adjust medications accordingly.

5. Inpatient management is indicated if the patient presents with fever (above 101°F), seizures, protracted nausea, vomiting, diarrhea, or signs of the Wernicke-Korsakoff syndrome.

6. Use a supportive approach for the anxious and perplexed patient. Reassurance and explanations may be helpful.

7. If the patient has a history of concomitant cocaine dependence, vital sign elevation may not be a reliable indication of withdrawal, as large amounts of cocaine may result in adrenergic depletion. In this case, alterations in mental status may be the best indication of withdrawal, and presumptive prophylaxis should be initiated.

8. Note: Heavy drinkers may begin withdrawing while their blood alcohol level remains elevated. These patients will not appear to be clinically intoxicated. Absolute blood alcohol level is not a reliable determinant of imminent withdrawal. Patients need to be observed clinically.

Medication and Nutrition

Benzodiazepines relieve the withdrawal, increase the seizure threshold, and provide adequate sedation. **Chlordiazepoxide 25 to 100 mg** should be prescribed as necessary for return or persistence of withdrawal symptoms. **Lorazepam 1 to 2 mg or diazepam (Valium) 10 to 20 mg** is an acceptable alternative. A single loading dose of **chlordiazepoxide 200 to 400 mg or diazepam 20 to 40 mg PRN** may be used. Lorazepam has a shorter half-life and predictable clearance and can be administered comfortably intramuscularly (IM), which may be an advantage for elderly or agitated patients or those with liver disease, chronic obstructive pulmonary disease, delirium, dementia, or other cognitive disorders.

Propranolol (Inderal) as an adjuvant to benzodiazepines has been shown to be of some use in reducing the severity of withdrawal and shortening hospital stay. Propranolol should not be given if the heart rate is less than 50. **Propranolol 50 mg** should be given to patients with a heart rate of 50 to 79. **Propranolol 100 mg** should be given to patients with a heart rate equal to or greater than 80. **Propranolol should be tapered by 60 mg a day until a dosage of 60 mg a day is reached. Thereafter, it should be tapered by 10 to 20 mg a day every 3 to 4 days.**

Indicated nutritional supplements include the following:

1. **Thiamine, 100 mg IM twice a day (BID) for the first 3 to 5 days and then PO to complete a course of 7 days.** (The first doses should be given IM because malabsorption is common in alcohol abusers.) Thiamine is essential to prevent the development of the Wernicke-Korsakoff syndrome.
2. **Folic acid, 1 mg PO every day (QD) for 7 days.**
3. **Vitamin B complex, 1 tablet PO QD for 7 days.**

Management of Seizures

Seizures occur in 5% to 15% of patients, are typically tonic-clonic, and are one or two in number. They usually develop within 6 to 48 hours but can also occur as late as 7 days following cessation of alcohol use. About 30% of patients who have seizures will develop withdrawal delirium.

Administer IV diazepam until seizure activity ceases. Give **IV diazepam 5 to 10 mg initially, and repeat if necessary at 10- to 15-minute intervals up to a maximum dose of 30 mg (inject slowly, taking at least 1 minute for each 5 mg given).**

Call a neurology consultation.

Phenytoin (Dilantin) should not be administered unless the patient has a known primary seizure disorder.

Management of Withdrawal Delirium

Withdrawal delirium (DTs) is a medical emergency. It occurs in less than 5% of individuals and usually begins 48 to 96 hours (or rarely 1 week) after cessation or decrease in alcohol intake. It usually occurs in individuals who have been drinking heavily for 5 to 15 years. If seizures also occur, they almost always precede the development of delirium. Withdrawal delirium may last 1 to 5 days. If untreated, mortality may be as high as 20%.

This potentially life-threatening condition includes disturbances in consciousness and cognition (e.g., disorientation, memory impairment); visual, tactile, or auditory hallucinations; agitation; and marked autonomic hyperactivity (e.g., tremulousness, tachycardia, hyperthermia, diaphoresis). It may lead to circulatory collapse, coma, and death. When alcohol withdrawal delirium develops, it is likely that a clinically related general medical condition may be present (e.g., liver failure, pneumonia, gastrointestinal bleeding, sequelae of head trauma, hypoglycemia, pancreatitis, an electrolyte imbalance, or postoperative status).

Follow the preceding guidelines for the management of uncomplicated withdrawal. In addition:

1. Secure an IV access.
2. **Lorazepam 2 mg or diazepam 10 mg may be given IM or IV if the oral route is not an option.** Doses should be repeated until symptoms clear. The total dosage given on the first day should be the standing dosage given on the second day. It should then be tapered gradually over the course of 3 to 4 days.
3. **Haloperidol 2 to 5 mg, IM or IV, every 2 to 4 hours** may be used to control severe cases of agitation or psychosis. It should be used with caution, however, as it may lower the seizure threshold and is metabolized hepatically.
4. Avoid physical restraints, if possible, as the patient may fight them and cause injury. Specifically, be alert to the possibility of sharp elevations in creatine phosphokinase (CPK) level.
5. Observe the patient closely for the development of focal neurologic signs.
6. Put the patient on a high-calorie, high-carbohydrate diet.

Other Complications

Other complications encountered during alcohol withdrawal include the Wernicke-Korsakoff syndrome and alcohol hallucinosis. Although they are not believed to be caused directly by alcohol withdrawal, they may complicate the clinical picture.

Wernicke's encephalopathy is an acute, potentially reversible neurologic disorder thought to be caused by thiamine deficiency. It is characterized by disturbances of consciousness (ranging from mild confusion to coma), ophthalmoplegia (sixth cranial nerve palsy), nystagmus, broad-based ataxia, peripheral neuropathy, hypothermia, and hypotension. It is usually seen in individuals with chronic heavy alcohol abuse and nutritional deficiencies. This disorder has a high mortality rate if untreated and can also progress to a more chronic condition known as **Korsakoff's psychosis.** Korsakoff's psychosis usually presents as a disturbance of short-term memory, inability to learn new information, and compensatory confabulation.

Alcoholic hallucinosis is characterized by vivid and persistent illusions and hallucinations with clear sensorium. The hallucinations and illusions may also affect the auditory and tactile modalities. This disorder may last several weeks or months. Antipsychotics may relieve agitation and hallucinations in those patients who do not improve spontaneously. **Haloperidol 2 to 5 mg PO or IM every 6 to 8 hours** may be used.

Sedative/Hypnotic/Anxiolytic Withdrawal

Warning: Withdrawal from central nervous system (CNS) depressants may be life threatening, and its treatment should precede the treatment of any other coexisting withdrawal syndromes. Adequate cardiac monitoring and ventilatory control should be available. Agents in this category include benzodiazepines, phenobarbital, pentobarbital, secobarbital, meprobamate, ethchlorvynol, glutethimide, chloral hydrate, and methaqualone. Withdrawal syndromes are likely to occur after chronic use of 40 to 60 mg per day of diazepam, 400 to 600 mg per day of pentobarbital, and 3200 to 6400 mg per day of meprobamate or their equivalents.

Signs and Symptoms

The signs and symptoms are essentially the same as those of alcohol withdrawal:

1. Autonomic hyperactivity (e.g., sweating, increased respirations, or pulse rate greater than 100)
2. Increased hand tremor
3. Insomnia
4. Nausea or vomiting
5. Transient visual, tactile, or auditory hallucinations or illusions with clear sensorium
6. Psychomotor agitation
7. Anxiety
8. Tonic-clonic seizures
9. Increased startle response
10. Increased deep tendon reflexes
11. Orthostatic hypotension

Time Course. The time of onset and duration of the sedative-hypnotic withdrawal syndrome depend largely on the pharmacokinetics of the particular agent. Initial symptoms may occur within 24 hours after the abstinence of a short-acting agent such as pentobarbital, but they may be delayed for as long as 1 week following abstinence from a longer-acting agent such as phenobarbital.

Immediate Steps

1. Order a tolerance test. The objective is to determine the starting dose for detoxification. Give the patient **pentobarbital (Nembutal) 200 mg.** Check 1 hour later:

a. If the patient is asleep, the tolerance dosage is **0 mg per day,** and no treatment for withdrawal is needed.
b. If the patient appears intoxicated and has coarse nystagmus, the tolerance dosage is **400 to 600 mg per day.**
c. If only fine nystagmus is present, the patient is tolerant to **800 mg per day.**
d. If no signs of intoxication appear, the patient is tolerant to **1200 mg per day** or more. Give an additional dose of **300 mg of pentobarbital 4 hours later.** If there is no change, the patient is tolerant to **1600 mg per day** or more.

2. Divide the above starting daily dose by four, and give every 6 hours for the first 2 days. Taper by 10% per day. Adjust according to signs of intoxication or withdrawal.
3. Note that equivalent medications are
   Phenobarbital 100 mg = pentobarbital 30 mg
   Diazepam 10 mg = pentobarbital 60 mg

Other Complications

Sedative, hypnotic, or anxiolytic withdrawal delirium can also occur. This potentially life-threatening condition includes disturbances in consciousness and cognition (e.g., disorientation, memory impairment); visual, tactile, or auditory hallucinations; agitation; and marked autonomic hyperactivity (e.g., tremulousness, tachycardia, hyperthermia, sweating). It may lead to circulatory collapse, coma, and death.

With the above presentations, especially when seen in the emergency room (ER), be sure to rule out metabolic, infectious, and structural abnormalities. Hypoglycemia and the Wernicke-Korsakoff syndrome must always be considered.

Opiate Withdrawal

Signs and Symptoms

In approximate order of appearance, the signs and symptoms of opiate withdrawal are

1. Anxiety, irritability, and craving
2. Dysphoric mood
3. Lacrimation and rhinorrhea
4. Insomnia
5. Yawning
6. Increased sensitivity to pain
7. Muscle, bone, and joint aches
8. Fever (usually low grade) and hot and cold flashes
9. Pupillary dilation, piloerection ("cold turkey"), and sweating
10. Nausea, vomiting, and diarrhea

11. Hyperadrenergic state: increased blood pressure, pulse, and respiratory rate
12. Muscle twitching and kicking ("kicking the habit")

Time Course.   Opioid withdrawal is characterized by anxiety, restlessness, aches often located in the back and legs, a wish to obtain opioids (craving), irritability, and increased sensitivity to pain. Tachycardia, hypertension, tachypnea, nausea, vomiting, diarrhea, and dehydration may occur in the most severe cases toward the peak of the withdrawal.

In most individuals who are dependent on short-acting drugs, such as heroin or morphine, withdrawal symptoms occur within 6 to 24 hours after the last dose. They peak at 48 to 72 hours and last 7 to 10 days. Symptoms may take 36 to 72 hours to emerge in the case of longer acting drugs, such as methadone or *l*-acetyl-α-methadol (LAAM).

Warning: In adults, the presence of high-grade fever, altered mental status, and seizures is inconsistent with opioid withdrawal and should alert the clinician to the possibility of another withdrawal syndrome (e.g., alcohol or sedative withdrawal), CNS infection, trauma, or sepsis.

Immediate Steps

Opioid withdrawal is uncomfortable but not life threatening. The objective in treating withdrawal is to reduce rather than suppress the symptoms. Patients should be told to expect some discomfort but be reassured that they will not be allowed to suffer or experience pain. The physician relies on objective findings (e.g., piloerection, sweating, rhinorrhea, pupillary changes, tachycardia, hypertension) to determine whether withdrawal is present; subjective complaints are less reliable as to the severity of the withdrawal. If the patient is enrolled in a methadone maintenance program, personnel from that program should be contacted to verify the daily dosage.

Medication

The main principle of treatment is replacement of the opioid agent. Methadone has become the replacement of choice in most cases because of its long half-life and ease of oral administration. If the patient's daily dosage can be verified through a methadone maintenance program, it can be safely given to the patient. If not, most patients in significant opioid withdrawal will have symptomatic relief with **5 to 10 mg of methadone initially,** regardless of the patient's daily intake of heroin or methadone. The advantage of such a dosage is that it can be given safely even to individuals who have never taken opioids without the risk of respiratory arrest. Consider IM administration because of its predictable absorption and efficacy despite the nausea, vomiting, and diarrhea commonly associated with opioid withdrawal, which may interfere with methadone absorption.

The methadone dose should be repeated every 4 to 6 hours until withdrawal symptoms disappear. **Total methadone intake during the first 24 hours should not exceed 40 mg** in most cases. The amount given the first day should be divided into two daily doses on the second day and then tapered at a rate of 10% to 20% per day.

Other opioid agents can be used in agonist substitution therapy:

1. LAAM is a longer acting preparation that can be administered less frequently than methadone (e.g., three times per week). It is usually prescribed in doses of **20 to 140 mg (average, 60 mg).**
2. Clonidine (Catapres) is an alpha$_2$-agonist antihypertensive agent that appears to be effective in alleviating insomnia, restlessness, nausea, vomiting, diarrhea, muscle aches, and craving associated with opioid withdrawal. As an adjunct to methadone treatment, it can help attenuate withdrawal and reduce its duration and cost. **Clonidine can be administered at 0.1 to 0.3 mg PO three or four times a day for 2 weeks. Do not exceed 0.8 mg a day.** The principal side effects are hypotension and sedation, and the dosage should be carefully individualized. Do not administer if the systolic blood pressure is less than 90 or the diastolic blood pressure is less than 60. Clonidine should be tapered on discontinuation because of the possibility of rebound hypertension.

Other Complications

Intravenous drug abusers may suffer from other medical complications of their habit. Be alert to possible signs and effects of endocarditis, trauma, intoxication with other substances, and malnutrition. The possibility of HIV and hepatitis C infection should also be considered.

CNS Stimulants (Cocaine and Amphetamine) Withdrawal

Signs and Symptoms

1. Depressed mood, which may be severe
2. Disturbing dreams
3. Fatigue, with sleep dysfunction
4. Increased appetite
5. Psychomotor retardation or agitation
6. Paranoid ideation

Time Course.   A triphasic pattern of behavior is described for cocaine withdrawal:

1. Crash phase (9 hours to 4 days after the last binge): This phase begins with agitation, depression, anorexia, and high drug craving. These are followed by a decrease in drug craving and by fatigue, depression, and a desire for sleep. Long periods of sleep are followed by intermittent periods of bulimia. The patient's sensorium is intact when awakened.
2. Withdrawal phase (1 to 10 weeks after the last binge): This phase begins with normalization of sleep and mood patterns, only to be followed again several days later by anhedonia, anergia, and anxiety, with high cocaine craving.
3. Extinction phase (may last for years): This phase represents a period of extended vulnerability to relapse, especially to conditioned cues.

Immediate Steps

The most acute problem in the management of both cocaine and amphetamine withdrawal is suicide. During the crash phase of withdrawal, patients may experience intense dysphoria and be at risk for impulsive suicide attempts. Although no factors are reliably predictive of the suicide potential, factors associated with an increased risk of suicide are male sex, single status, age in the 40- to 60-year range, lack of social and familial support systems, recent discharge from psychiatric hospitalization, previous suicide attempts, and alcoholism.

Suicidal patients may require admission to the hospital or at least be re-evaluated in 24 hours. Patients should be encouraged to attend a detoxification or rehabilitation program and referred to a support group, such as Narcotics Anonymous (NA). Family or group therapy can also be helpful.

Medication

Lorazepam 1 to 2 mg, PO or IM, can be given to control agitation and maladaptive behavior. If paranoid ideation is present to a significant extent, antipsychotics, such as **haloperidol (Haldol) 5 to 10 mg PO or IM** or its equivalent, can be added.

Desipramine (Norpramin) has been considered of possible, although limited, use in treating the dysphoria and drug craving. The usual starting dose is **75 mg.** After several days, it can be gradually titrated to **200 to 300 mg.** It has also been proposed that cocaine induces a state of relative dopaminergic deficiency. Bromocriptine (Parlodel), amantadine (Symmetrel), and the dopamine precursor tyrosine have been reported to reduce cocaine craving in the first week or two after withdrawal. The potential of these agents to aggravate a paranoid psychotic state should, however, be kept in mind.

Remember: A substantial number of individuals with cocaine dependence have few or no clinically evident withdrawal symptoms upon cessation of use.

Nicotine Withdrawal

Signs and Symptoms

Nicotine withdrawal will be commonly encountered as a by-product of hospitalization in a nonsmoking facility. The withdrawal syndrome includes four or more of the following:

1. Dysphoric or depressed mood
2. Insomnia
3. Irritability, frustration, or anger
4. Anxiety
5. Difficulty concentrating
6. Restlessness
7. Decreased heart rate
8. Increased appetite or weight gain

Time Course.   Typically the sense of craving peaks within 24 hours and then declines gradually over a period of 10 days to several weeks. As with cocaine and other drugs, however, craving can be powerfully evoked by cues previously associated with smoking or tobacco use.

Medication

Nicotine replacement therapy with transdermal nicotine (TN), a nicotine inhaler, or **nicotine polacrilex (Nicorette gum 2 mg or DS, 9 to 12 pieces per day)** doubles long-term abstinence rates (from 4% to 8%). When combined with behavioral therapy, success rates of up to 40% have been reported. It is important to ensure that the patient does not smoke while undergoing replacement therapy, as nicotine overdose can occur.

Clonidine (Catapres) has also been effective in alleviating withdrawal symptoms but appears to be less effective than TN. **Start at 0.1 mg BID with daily increments of 0.1 mg** until the desired response is achieved. Do not give more than **0.8 mg** per day.

Compliance with long-term smoking cessation can be supported with the initiation of buproprion (Zyban). This should be initiated only with patients who are motivated to quit smoking.

Antidepressant Withdrawal

Signs and Symptoms

1. Nausea, vomiting, diarrhea, and abdominal pain
2. Malaise
3. Myalgias
4. Fatigue

5. Hot flashes and diaphoresis
6. Anxiety
7. Insomnia

Less common symptoms may include movement disorders, such as akathisia and parkinsonism, or psychiatric symptoms such as hypomania, mania, and panic attacks.

Immediate Steps

The treatment of antidepressant withdrawal, if severe, is to reinstitute the antidepressant and then taper the drug gradually. Minor symptoms usually abate spontaneously. Discontinuation of an antidepressant with a short half-life (e.g., paroxetine) is more likely to precipitate withdrawal than is an agent with a longer half-life (e.g., fluoxetine). Fluoxetine may be used for a patient withdrawing from a short–half-life selective serotonin reuptake inhibitor, as it will self-taper.

Anticholinergic Drug Withdrawal

Signs and Symptoms

Withdrawal symptoms usually resemble those of influenza. Anticholinergic drugs may occasionally produce depressed mood, manic-like symptoms, or seizures when withdrawn abruptly. Reinstitution of the medication and gradual tapering are the mainstays of treatment.

19 | Insomnia

SEAN ALLAN

Insomnia is frequently a symptom of another disorder. The key to treating insomnia is to search for the underlying cause. As with any consultation, each patient deserves a complete evaluation and appropriate treatment. You may be tempted to quickly prescribe sedating medications for patients complaining of sleeplessness, especially when you would like to be asleep yourself. Beware of medicating patients for insomnia, however, without first assessing them. This will avoid mistreating people with hidden medical, psychiatric, or more serious sleep disorders.

Insomnia is the complaint of insufficient sleep associated with adverse daytime consequences such as anergy, malaise, cognitive slowness, and irritability. Insomnia is best understood as a symptom with numerous potential underlying causes. Mild transient sleep disturbance secondary to anxiety or physical discomfort is very common in hospitalized patients. If the patient has no daytime compromise in functioning, you can monitor the insomnia and defer treatment with hypnotics.

■ PHONE CALL

Questions

1. Who is requesting help, the patient or the staff?
2. What is the patient's admission diagnosis, and when was he or she admitted to the hospital?
3. Is the patient also anxious, agitated, or acting strangely?

    Remember, a patient who is sleepless and agitated or acting bizarrely requires prompt evaluation.
4. Has the patient had complaints of insomnia previous to this hospitalization or this consult? If so, what forms of treatment were suggested? Were these beneficial to the patient?
5. Has there been any recent change in the patient's clinical status or medications?

Orders

If the patient is well known to you, is not in acute distress, and has a history of difficulty initiating or maintaining sleep that responded well to medication in the past, you may consider renewing the medication order. If the patient is not familiar to you, resist the temptation to issue a telephone order and go assess the patient.

Inform RN

"Will arrive in . . . minutes."

Remember

A patient who is sleepless and agitated or acting bizarrely requires prompt evaluation. Also refer to Chapter 8 on the agitated patient.

■ ELEVATOR THOUGHTS

What causes insomnia?
    The etiology will often be readily identified by assessing the onset, duration, and nature of the patient's sleep complaint.
1. **Environmental and behavioral factors**
    a. Unpleasant or noisy sleep environment
    b. Situational anxiety
    c. Preoccupation with falling asleep
    d. Disrupted circadian rhythm (e.g., shift work or jet lag)
2. **Psychiatric and neurologic disorders**
    a. Affective disorders (e.g., depression or mania)
    b. Anxiety disorders (e.g., adjustment disorder with anxiety features, obsessive-compulsive disorder, panic attacks, post-traumatic stress disorder)
    c. Psychosis (intrusive hallucinations or paranoia)
    d. Akathisia
    e. Dementia
    f. Neurodegenerative disorders (e.g., Parkinson's disease)
3. **Substance abuse and withdrawal symptoms**
4. **Medications, including caffeine and nicotine**
5. **Related medical problems**

■ MAJOR THREAT TO LIFE

- Overmedication or inappropriate medication with sedatives
- Unrecognized medical problem manifesting as insomnia
- Undiagnosed obstructive or central sleep apnea syndrome

■ BEDSIDE

Remember that your task here is to distinguish symptoms of benign sleeplessness from occult conditions that require further evaluation and for which a sedating medication may be contraindicated (Table 19–1)

Quick Look Test

Is the patient in bed or wandering?

Does the patient look uncomfortable or anxious?

Does the patient seem manipulative or demanding?

Is the patient exhibiting tachycardia, hypertension, or fever?

Is there a trend in the patient's vital signs that would indicate an occult illness (e.g., uncontrolled hypertension or withdrawal states)?

Selective Chart Review

1. When and why was the patient admitted?
   - Recently admitted patients may have difficulty sleeping owing to the new environment or to new medications. Alternatively, the patient may have an underlying chronic, unrecognized sleep disturbance.
   - Patients who have been hospitalized for a while may develop disturbed circadian rhythms secondary to frequent daytime naps and disruptions from nighttime sleep (e.g., for vital sign measurements or blood work or because of neighboring patients).
2. Is there a history of substance abuse?
   - Sleeplessness may be one of the first signs of acute withdrawal states from alcohol, narcotics, or benzodiazepines. Withdrawal states may become life threatening (see Chapter 18).
   - Recovering substance abusers may sleep poorly for months to years after cessation of drinking or illicit drug

Table 19–1 □ CONTRAINDICATIONS TO SEDATIVE-HYPNOTIC MEDICATIONS

Hepatic or respiratory failure
Delirium or confusion
Sleep apnea
Myasthenia gravis
Concomitant use of alcohol or narcotics (potentiation)

use. Heavy nicotine dependence frequently leads to a nighttime withdrawal syndrome of frequent awakenings to smoke cigarettes.

3. What are the patient's age, sex, and current medical and psychiatric status?
   - Pay special attention to medical problems that may make the patient uncomfortable.
   - Elderly patients have a greater incidence of occult primary sleep disorders and a greater predisposition for disturbed sleep owing to medications and medical or psychiatric disorders.
4. Were sleep complaints made or were sleep disorders observed previously? If so, what treatments were attempted, and which were successful?

Selective History

The sleep history should include a general characterization of the severity, duration, variability, and daytime consequences of sleep deprivation.

Common questions to ask include the following:

1. When did your insomnia begin?
2. Do you have difficulty primarily in falling asleep, staying asleep, waking too early, or a combination? How long are you typically awake before falling asleep again?

   Anxiety, environmental noise, or physical discomfort (especially **pain**) can make it difficult to fall asleep. A variety of intrinsic sleep and psychiatric disorders can lead to problems in maintaining sleep at night. Remember to ask the patient what he or she perceives as the cause of the multiple awakenings. Also, ask about nightmares with early awakenings, restlessness, leg "kicking" or cramping in the limbs, and loud snoring with gasping or choking upon awakening (collateral sources of information can be helpful with these questions).

3. Are you sleepy during the day? Do you nap?

   Remember that a diagnosis of insomnia includes daytime sleepiness as well as decreased perception of sleep at night. Does the patient complain of fatigue, difficulty in completing tasks, mood symptoms, irritability, or concentration problems?

3. Do you drink caffeine or alcohol? Do you use benzodiazepines or narcotics? Do you smoke cigarettes?
4. Do you have any other symptoms of psychiatric illness (e.g., depression, anxiety, obsessive-compulsive disorder, psychosis, dementia, or delirium)?

■ COMMON CAUSES OF INSOMNIA

Medical Problems

Some common medical problems that cause insomnia are listed in Tables 19–2 and 19–3. Chronic insomnia may be a symptom of a disease in virtually any organ or a side effect of medication. It is preferable to relieve the insomnia associated with a chronic medical condition by specifically treating the condition itself. Only when there is no accepted treatment for the primary medical

Table 19–2 □ COMMON MEDICAL CAUSES OF INSOMNIA

Neurologic disorders
1. Stroke
   a. Increased incidence of obstructive sleep apnea, central sleep apnea, or periodic limb movement disorder
   b. Increased incidence of depression after stroke
2. Alzheimer's disease—in later stages is associated with circadian rhythm disorder
3. Parkinson's disease—associated with parasomnias (e.g., rapid eye movement [REM] behavior disorder) and insomnia
4. Chronic pain—produces difficulty in initiating and maintaining sleep

Cardiovascular disease
1. Nocturnal angina pectoris
2. Congestive heart failure (CHF)
   a. Supine posture redistributes blood to the central circulatory system, worsening paroxysmal nocturnal dyspnea
   b. CHF is accompanied by Cheyne-Stokes respiration, leading to repeated awakenings
   3. Hypertension—insomnia may be caused by uncontrolled hypertension or may be secondary to use of antihypertensive medications

Pulmonary disease*
1. Chronic obstructive pulmonary disease (COPD). Note: Nasal canula O_2 reduces sleep-onset latency, increases the duration of uninterrupted sleep, and improves nocturnal oxygen saturation in this population
2. Asthma

Gastrointestinal disorders
1. Gastroesophageal reflux disease (GERD)—symptoms can occur only during sleep or can significantly worsen during sleep

Endocrine disorders
1. Thyroid disorders
2. Diabetes mellitus—may be related to hyperglycemia, hypoglycemia, nocturia, or pain from peripheral neuropathy
3. Perimenopause—insomnia may respond to hormone replacement therapy
4. Obesity

*Drug therapies for COPD and asthma, including methylxanthines, oral beta-agonists, and oral glucocorticoids, can also cause insomnia.

Table 19–3 □ POSSIBLE IATROGENIC CAUSES OF INSOMNIA

Antiasthmatics: beta₂-agonists, theophylline
Anticonvulsants: phenytoin, carbamazepine, valproic acid
Antidepressants: phenelzine, tranylcypromine, protriptyline,
    desipramine, imipramine, amoxapine, selective serotonin reuptake
    inhibitors, tricyclic withdrawal, venlafaxine, bupropion
Antihypertensives: beta-blockers, methyldopa, diuretics, reserpine,
    clonidine
Antipsychotics: phenothiazines, butyrophenones
Cimetidine
Decongestants: pseudoephedrine, phenylephrine
Levodopa, baclofen, methylsergide
Sedative-hypnotics (rebound insomnia), barbiturates,
    benzodiazepines, narcotics
Stimulants: amphetamines, methylphenidate, pemoline
Tetracycline
Thyroxine, steroids, birth control pills

condition or when treatment of the medical condition fails to alleviate the insomnia should the consultant treat only the symptom.

Psychiatric Disorders

Psychiatric disorders are the leading cause of chronic insomnia (Table 19–4). Insomnia is a symptom of major depression, dysthymia, mania, and anxiety disorders but can also be a component of psychosis, dementia, and substance abuse or withdrawal.

Primary Sleep Disorders

- Restless legs syndrome (during wakefulness, a sensation of unpleasant pulling or drawing deep in the muscles of the

Table 19–4 □ PSYCHIATRIC CAUSES OF INSOMNIA

Anxiety disorders
Affective disorders
Dementia
Psychosis (neuroleptic-induced akathisia or night-day reversal in
    paranoid schizophrenics)
Substance intoxication (stimulants, amphetamines, cocaine,
    "Ecstasy," nicotine)
Substance withdrawal (caffeine, alcohol, nicotine, benzodiazepines)

lower extremities that worsens in the evening hours). Symptoms decrease with dopamine agonists (e.g., levodopa/carbidopa, pergolide) or bedtime doses of clonazepam.

- Periodic limb movement disorder (during sleep, movement of limbs that may be accompanied by electroencephalographic [EEG] arousal, disturbing the continuity of sleep). Treatment is the same as for restless legs syndrome.

- Obstructive sleep apnea (repetitive closure of the upper airway during sleep, resulting in increased labor of breathing accompanied by multiple arousals from sleep). Loud snoring with choking or gasping occurs. Treatment is continuous positive airway pressure (CPAP), use of a dental appliance, or upper airway surgery. Obstructive sleep apnea requires evaluation in a sleep laboratory or by an ear, nose, and throat (ENT) specialist.

- Central sleep apnea (repetitive loss of respiratory drive, leading to a cyclic fluctuation in respiratory effort, EEG arousal, and disturbance of sleep continuity). Consultation should by assisted by a pulmonary specialist.

Poor Sleep Hygiene

Poor sleep hygiene insomnia results from sleep-incompatible behaviors just before or throughout bedtime. Such behaviors include exercising or eating close to bedtime, not allowing for "winding down" time before bedtime, and failing to protect the sleeping environment from adverse temperatures and avoidable sources of noise (e.g., television).

■ MANAGEMENT

Successful treatment of insomnia alleviates nighttime complaints without compromising daytime functioning. Medication

Table 19–5 □ IMPORTANT ELEMENTS OF GOOD SLEEP HYGIENE

Quiet, comfortable environment
No stimulants, alcohol, heavy meals, or vigorous exercise within 3 to 4 hours before bedtime
Moderate exercise earlier than 4 hours before bedtime
No daytime naps
Regular wake time
Reinforce waking hours with exposure to light early in the day and physical activity if possible
Address life stressors and any obsessive concerns regarding ability to sleep

Table 19–6 □ COGNITIVE/BEHAVIORAL APPROACHES TO INSOMNIA

1. Do not go to bed until sleepy
2. Lie in bed only when attempting to sleep
3. If unable to sleep, get out of bed
4. Use relaxation techniques to decrease anxiety
   a. Progressive muscle relaxation
   b. Visualization
   c. Correct negative thoughts, e.g., "I didn't sleep last night, so I won't be able to sleep tonight."
   d. Avoid catastrophic thoughts, e.g., "I'll die if I don't get a good night's sleep."
   e. Insert positive thoughts

Table 19–7 □ ADJUNCT MEDICATION TO TREAT INSOMNIA

Benzodiazepines* (should be used at their lowest effective dose and only for acute complaints of insomnia)
Alprazolam (Xanax) 0.25–0.5 mg PO QHS ($t_{1/2}$ = 12 h)
Lorezapam (Ativan) 0.5–2 mg PO QHS ($t_{1/2}$ = 10–20 h)
Temazepam (Restoril) 7.5–30 mg PO QHS ($t_{1/2}$ = 8–25 h)
Novel benzodiazepine-receptor agonists†
Zolpidem tartrate (Ambien) 5–10 mg PO QHS ($t_{1/2}$ =2.5 h)
Zaleplon (Sonata) 5–10 mg PO QHS ($t_{1/2}$ = 1 h)
Sedating antidepressants (indicated for depressed/anxious patients)
Trazodone (Desyrel) 25–150 mg PO QHS
Doxepin (Sinequan) 25–50 mg PO QHS
Nefazodone (Serzone) 100–300 mg PO QHS
Mirtazapine (Remeron) 15–30 mg PO QHS; 15 mg is more sedating
Antihistamines‡
Diphenhydramine hydrochloride (Benadryl) 50 mg PO QHS
Hydroxyzine hydrochloride (Atarax/Vistaril) 25–100 mg PO QHS
Sedating antipsychotics§ (indicated for patients with psychosis, mania, or cognitive impairment/sundowning)
Thioridazine (Mellaril) 10–50 mg PO QHS
Haloperidol (Haldol) 2–5 mg PO QHS (0.5–2 mg for sundowning)

$t_{1/2}$ = half-life.
*Potential for recreational abuse, increased risk of falls, delayed reaction time, increased risk of machinery accidents, residual morning sedation, rebound insomnia, anterograde amnesia, tolerance, and dependence.
†Tolerance, dependence, and withdrawal syndromes unclear.
‡Potential for morning sedation, dry mucous membranes, risk of anticholinergic delirium.
§Potential for inducing akathisia.

treatment of secondary insomnia should be evaluated on a case-by-case basis. Use of hypnotic agents should be recommended only after the primary cause has been evaluated. The ideal hypnotic would be completely absorbed, undergo minimal first-pass hepatic metabolism, be rapidly transferred from blood to brain, be completely metabolized by the end of sleep time, and be associated with minimal tolerance and dependence.

1. Evaluate, address, and treat underlying causes of insomnia.
2. Evaluate and recommend changes in sleep hygiene (Table 19–5)
3. Recommend cognitive/behavioral approaches (Table 19–6)
4. Evaluate need for adjunct sedative-hypnotic medication (Table 19–7). Select a medicine that also treats an underlying Axis I or II disorder.

20 | Headache

MADELEINE CASTELLANOS

Headaches are a common complaint on a psychiatric service and may be a symptom of a serious medical condition or a manifestation of a psychiatric disorder, such as anxiety or depression, or of emotional stress. It is important to evaluate the patient's complaint and to determine whether the headache is of no urgent concern or is a symptom of a more serious condition.

■ PHONE CALL

Questions

1. **How severe is the headache?**
    Most headaches are mild and not of major concern unless associated with other symptoms.
2. **Was the onset sudden or gradual?**
    The sudden onset of a severe headache is suggestive of a subarachnoid hemorrhage, or it may indicate a hypertensive crisis in a patient taking monoamine oxidase inhibitors (MAOIs), e.g., phenelzine, tranylcypromine.
3. **What are the current vital signs and the baseline values?**
4. **Has there been a change in the level of consciousness?**
5. **Does the patient have a history of chronic or recurrent headaches?**
6. **What are the patient's diagnoses?**
7. **What medications is the patient taking?**

Orders

1. Ask the nurse for vital signs (blood pressure, heart rate, temperature) if they have not been recorded in the last 30 minutes.
2. If the headache is mild and you are confident that it represents a previously diagnosed recurrent problem, it may be appropriate to prescribe a non-narcotic analgesic (e.g., acetaminophen or ibuprofen). If you cannot see the patient immediately because of other emergencies, ask the nurse to call back in 1 to 2 hours if the headache has not been relieved by the medication.

Inform RN

"Will arrive in . . . minutes."

If the patient's headache is associated with fever, vomiting, or an altered mental status or if he or she has a severe headache with an acute onset, you need to see the patient immediately. An assessment at the bedside is also necessary if the headache is more severe than usual for the patient or if the character of the pain is different from usual.

■ ELEVATOR THOUGHTS

What are causes of chronic (recurrent) headaches?
1. Muscle contraction
   a. Tension headaches secondary to depression, anxiety, stress
   b. Cervical osteoarthritis
   c. Temporomandibular joint disease
2. Vascular
   a. Migraine
   b. Cluster headaches
3. Drugs/withdrawal
   a. Nitrates
   b. Calcium channel blockers
   c. Acquired immunodeficiency syndrome (AIDS) medications
   d. Caffeine, nicotine, alcohol, or illicit drug withdrawal
4. Referred pain
   a. Toothache
   b. Dental abcess

What are causes of acute headache?
1. Infections
   a. Meningitis
   b. Encephalitis
   c. Viremia
2. Post-trauma
   a. Concussion
   b. Cerebral contusion
   c. Subdural or epidural hematoma
3. Vascular
   a. Subarachnoid hemorrhage
   b. Intracerebral hemorrhage
   c. Arteriovenous malformation
   d. Cerebral infarction
4. Increased intracranial pressure
   a. Space-occupying lesions
   b. Malignant hypertension (hypertensive crisis)
   c. Benign intracranial hypertension

5. Local causes
    a. Temporal arteritis
    b. Acute angle-closure glaucoma

■ MAJOR THREAT TO LIFE

- **Subarachnoid hemorrhage** is associated with a very high mortality rate if left untreated.
- **Bacterial meningitis** must be recognized early if antibiotic treatment is to be successful.
- **Herniation** (transtentorial, cerebellar, central) may occur as a result of a tumor, a subdural or epidural hematoma, or any other mass lesion.
- **Hypertensive crisis** may result from the interaction of MAOIs and tyramine-containing foods or sympathomimetic drugs and requires immediate control of blood pressure to prevent consequences.

■ BEDSIDE

Quick Look Test

Does the patient look well (comfortable), sick (uncomfortable), or critical?

Most patients with chronic headache appear well. Those with severe migraines, subarachnoid hemorrhage, meningitis, or hypertensive crisis appear sick.

Vital Signs

What is the patient's temperature?

When a fever is associated with a headache, you must decide whether a lumbar puncture (LP) should be performed to rule out meningitis.

What is the patient's blood pressure?

A sudden and dramatic increase in blood pressure (BP) associated with a severe occipital headache, a stiff neck, sweating, nausea, and vomiting in a patient taking MAOIs signifies a hypertensive crisis. Malignant hypertension (hypertension with papilledema) is usually associated with a systolic BP of more than 190 mm Hg and a diastolic BP of more than 120 mm Hg. Headaches usually do not occur as a symptom of hypertension unless there has been a recent increase in pressure.

What is the patient's heart rate?

Hypertension in association with bradycardia may be a manifestation of increasing intracranial pressure.

Selective History and Chart Review

1. Onset

   The abrupt onset of a severe headache suggests a vascular cause, the most serious being subarachnoid or intracerebral hemorrhage.

2. Severity

   Most muscle contraction headaches are not incapacitating. However, migraine headaches are associated with severe pain, and the patient might look quite sick.

3. Position

   Most muscle contraction headaches are improved by lying down. Headaches that are worse in the supine position suggest increased intracranial pressure, and an intracranial mass should be considered.

4. History of recent trauma

   An epidural hematoma may occur after even a relatively minor head injury, particularly in teenagers or young adults. Subdural hematomas can appear insidiously (6 to 8 weeks) after a seemingly mild head trauma and are not uncommonly seen in the alcoholic patient.

5. History of procedures

   An LP is often followed by a headache appearing several hours to 1 day after the procedure. The incidence is higher when a large-bore needle is used or if several punctures are performed. This type of headache is usually bifrontal or generalized and is worse when the patient sits upright. It is believed to be caused by intracranial hypotension due to CSF loss, which results in displacement of pain-sensitive structures when the patient is upright. The patient may experience relief when lying flat (prone or supine).

6. Visual changes

   Acute angle-closure glaucoma can be precipitated by pupillary dilatation. The patient commonly complains of a severe unilateral headache located over the brow, which may be accompanied by nausea, vomiting, and abdominal pain.

7. Prodromal symptoms

   Nausea and vomiting are associated with increased intracranial pressure but may also occur with migraines or angle-closure glaucoma. Photophobia and neck stiffness are associated with meningitis. Typical prodromal symptoms of a migraine include nausea, vomiting, photophobia, visual

scotomata, geometric visual phenomena, and unilateral
paresthesias and may be helpful in making the diagnosis.

8. MAOIs

Headache accompanied by a stiff neck, sweating, nausea,
or vomiting in a patient taking MAOIs may signify a hypertensive crisis secondary to the ingestion of tyramine-containing foods and is a medical emergency requiring immediate pharmacologic intervention (Table 20–1).

9. Other medications

Drugs such as nitrates, calcium channel blockers, and
nonsteroidal anti-inflammatory drugs (NSAIDs) can cause
headaches.

10. History of caffeine, nicotine, alcohol, or other drug use

Acute withdrawal from any of these substances can cause
headaches. Be especially aware of the heavy smoker who
is placed in the hospital, usually a nonsmoking environment, and forced to acutely stop smoking.

11. Temporomandibular joint (TMJ) dysfunction

Patients who experience any clicking or popping when
operating or closing the jaw, or who grind their teeth at

Table 20–1 □ MAOI DIETARY RESTRICTION OF TYRAMINE-CONTAINING FOODS

Must Be Avoided
Most cheese and cheese products
Fermented meats (sausage, salami, pepperoni)
Aged meats
Liver
Smoked or pickled herring
Caviar
Sauerkraut
Yeast extract or dietary supplements (brewer's
  yeast, "Marmite," some packaged soups)
Chianti wine
Vermouth
Acceptable in Moderate Amounts
Sour cream
Yogurt
Avocado
Bananas
Tomatoes
Raisins
Spinach
Soy sauce
Beers
Ales

Modified from Keller MB, Boland RJ: Antidepressants. In Tasman A, Kay J, Lieberman JA (eds): Psychiatry. Philadelphia, WB Saunders, 1997, p 1622.

night or wake with mandibular tension, may be suffering from TMJ dysfunction. These patients may report pain predominantly in the ear or face.

12. Joint disease in the neck or upper back

Muscle contraction headaches in the elderly are often caused by cervical osteoarthritis. These headaches characteristically start in the neck region and radiate to the temple or the forehead.

13. History of chronic (recurrent) headaches

Migraine and muscle contraction headaches follow a pattern. It is important to ask the patient if this headache is the same as a "usual" headache.

14. Psychiatric diagnosis

The somatoform disorders (somatization disorder, conversion disorder, hypochondriasis, pain disorder) are a group of disorders that include physical symptoms for which no adequate medical explanation can be found. Nonpsychiatric medical causes must always be ruled out before a psychiatric diagnosis can be made. For patients with a somatoform, disorder, the complaint of headache should always be taken seriously, and your approach should be a supportive one.

Selective Physical Examination

1. Head, eyes, ears, nose, and throat (HEENT)
   a. Nuchal rigidity (meningitis or subarachnoid hemorrhage)
   b. Papilledema (increased intracranial pressure) (Fig. 20–1 shows the funduscopic features of papilledema)
   c. Red eye (acute angle-closure glaucoma)
   d. Hemotympanum, or blood in the ear canal (basal skull fracture)
   e. Tender, enlarged temporal arteries (temporal arteritis)
   f. Retinal hemorrhages (hypertension)
   g. Lid ptosis, dilated pupil, eye deviated down and out (posterior communicating cerebral artery aneurysm)
   h. Tenderness on palpation or failure of transillumination of the frontal and maxillary sinuses (sinusitis or subdural hematoma)
   i. Inability to fully open the jaw (temporomandibular joint [TMJ] dysfunction)
2. Neurologic
   a. Mental status changes and altered level of consciousness may accompany meningitis, intracranial hemorrhage, electrolyte and metabolic disturbances, or complicated alcohol withdrawal
   b. Drowsiness, yawning, and inattentiveness associated with a

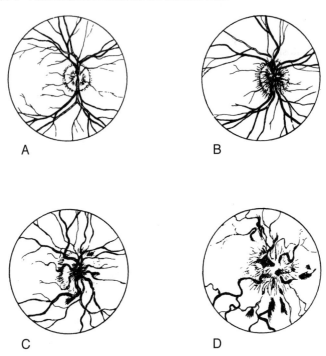

Figure 20-1 □ Disc changes seen in papilledema. **A.** Normal. **B.** Early papilledema. **C.** Moderate papilledema with early hemorrhage. **D.** Severe papilledema with extensive hemorrhage. (From Marshall SA, Ruedy J: On Call: Principles and Protocols. Philadelphia, WB Saunders, 1993, p. 104.)

      headache all are ominous signs and may be the only signs evident in a patient with a small subarachnoid hemorrhage

c. Asymmetric pupils associated with rapidly decreasing level of consciousness can represent a life-threatening situation. Call for a neurosurgical consult immediately to assess for probable uncal herniation.

d. Asymmetry of pupils, visual fields, eye movements, limbs, tone, reflexes, or plantar responses suggests structural brain disease. If this is a new finding, a computed tomographic (CT) scan or magnetic resonance imaging (MRI) of the head is necessary.

e. Kernig's sign (pain or resistance on passive knee extension from the 90° hip/knee flexion position) is an indication of possible meningitis

f. Brudzinski's sign (flexion of hips or knees in response to

passive neck flexion) is present with meningitis or subarachnoid hemorrhage
3. Musculoskeletal
   a. Palpate the skull and face looking for fractures, hematomas,
   and lacerations. Evidence of recent head trauma suggests
   the possibility of a subdural or an epidural hematoma.

■ MANAGEMENT

Serious Conditions

Bacterial Meningitis.   Meningitis should be suspected if there
is a headache accompanied by fever, nuchal rigidity, Kernig's or
Brudzinski's sign, and/or signs of cerebral dysfunction (confusion, delirium, or a decreasing level of consciousness, ranging
from lethargy to coma). Shaking chills, profuse sweating, photophobia, weakness, nausea, vomiting, anorexia, and myalgias are
also common findings. An immediate CT scan and lumbar puncture (LP) are indicated. Consult the medicine service regarding
antibiotics and further management of meningitis. Signs of increased intracranial pressure can develop later in the disease
course and carry a grave prognosis. A subdural empyema or a
brain abscess may cause nuchal rigidity and increased intracranial
pressure. If there is any sign of increased intracranial pressure
(papilledema, focal neurologic signs, or obtundation), an LP
would be contraindicated because of the risk of brain herniation.

Space-Occupying Lesions and Hemorrhages.   When an LP is
contraindicated, a CT scan will help identify an intracranial mass
or any obstruction to cerebrospinal fluid (CSF) outflow. Neurosur-
gery should be consulted immediately for any patients with subdural, epidural, or subarachnoid hemorrhage or with space-occupying lesions (brain abscess, tumor) causing raised intracranial
pressure.

Hypertensive Crisis.   Hypertensive crisis requires immediate
reduction in BP by the administration of **labetolol IV given as a
20- to 40-mg bolus, which may be repeated after 10 minutes.**
Alternatively, oral medications may be used, such as **captopril 25
mg, labetolol 200 mg,** or **clonidine 0.1 mg.** The patient should
be moved to a medical service. Call for a medical consultation
immediately.

Malignant Hypertension.   Malignant hypertension (hypertension and papilledema) should be managed by careful reduction
of BP. The medical service should be consulted for management
of this condition.

Glaucoma.   A patient with acute angle-closure glaucoma
should be referred to an ophthalmologist immediately.

Less Serious Conditions

Muscle Contraction Headaches.   Chronic muscle contraction headaches may be symptomatically treated with non-narcotic analgesics. This is the most common type of headache you will see in the hospital. Psychiatric patients are particularly susceptible to them, as they can be brought on by emotional stress and frequently occur in anxiety and depressive disorders. A long-term treatment plan, if not already established, may be discussed with the treatment team.

Migraine Headaches.   Mild migraines can be treated adequately with aspirin or acetaminophen. More severe migraines will respond best if treatment is initiated during the prodromal stage; however, it is unlikely that you will be called until the headache is well established. Ask the patient what he or she usually takes for migraine headaches, as that will probably be the most effective agent for that patient. A severe migraine often requires a narcotic analgesic agent, such as **codeine 30 to 60 mg orally or intramuscularly (IM) every 4 to 5 hours PRN** or **meperidine 50 to 100 mg IM every 3 to 4 hours PRN**.

Cluster Headaches.   Cluster headaches are difficult to treat. Most resolve spontaneously within 45 minutes, and oral treatment has minimal effect. Many patients gain partial relief when administered oxygen by nasal canula (2 L). If a cluster headache develops in the hospital and is severe, a parenteral narcotic may be tried, such as **codeine 30 to 60 mg IM** or **meperidine 50 to 100 mg IM**. Alternatively, **dihydroergotamine 0.75 mg intravenously (IV) now and repeated in 30 minutes** may be effective.

Postconcussion Headaches.   Postconcussion headaches (provided that subdural and epidural hemorrhages have been ruled out) should be treated with an analgesic agent that is unlikely to cause sedation (e.g., acetaminophen, codeine). Aspirin or NSAIDs are contraindicated for the post-trauma patient because the inhibition of platelet aggregation may predispose the patient to bleeding complications.

Benign Intracranial Hypertension.   Benign intracranial hypertension (pseudotumor cerebri) is a syndrome of unknown etiology, with increased intracranial pressure (headache and papilledema) and no evidence of a mass lesion or hydrocephalus. Refer the patient to a neurologist for further evaluation.

21 | Chest Pain

IRA L. SCOTT, JR.

While on call you may frequently be asked to see patients experiencing chest pain. Although chest pain has numerous causes, ranging from esophageal reflux to myocardial infarction, you should always assume that you are dealing with a life-threatening disorder until proved otherwise. Chest pain may be the initial indication of an impending medical emergency, so it is crucial that it be addressed quickly. This chapter focuses on problems most commonly encountered on the psychiatric ward. A calm and systematic approach, including a thorough history, will often provide most of the essential information necessary to make a correct diagnosis and lead you to appropriate management.

■ PHONE CALL

Questions

1. **What are the patient's vital signs, and have these changed?**
2. **Is the patient dyspneic or tachypneic?**
3. **When did the pain begin? How does the patient describe it?**
4. **Does the patient have a history of cardiovascular disease (myocardial infarction [MI], coronary artery disease [CAD], angina), reflux, or peptic ulcer disease?**
5. **Has the patient had any recent surgery, procedures, or drug use?**

Orders

It is best to assume that a serious medical condition (e.g., myocardial ischemia, MI, pulmonary embolism) is the cause of the pain until proved otherwise. Therefore, a good first rule is that all patients with chest pain should have an immediate electrocardiogram (ECG). This creates a permanent record of cardiac activity at the time of pain that is useful for

1. Assessing the heart's electrophysiologic status for ST segment, Q wave, and T wave changes and rhythm disturbances

2. Comparing with a prior ECG (presumably done on admission or in the past while the patient was not in distress)
3. Consulting with other physicians (e.g., a cardiologist) who might be called in later

A nurse should be asked to start an ECG while you are on your way to the ward. If no one is available to start the ECG, ask to have the machine set up and ready for your arrival in order to begin the assessment more quickly.

It is usually best to evaluate the patient personally before ordering medications. A patient with a known history of angina or other cardiac disease or who has been treated with nitroglycerin in the past may be given **0.4 mg sublingual nitroglycerin every 5 minutes up to three times** before your arrival (hold for systolic blood pressure <90 mm Hg). With the goal of preventing further possible coronary artery thrombus formation, have the patient **chew and swallow one 325-mg aspirin tablet.**

If the patient is reported as dyspneic or has had recent chest surgery, trauma, or invasive procedure (chest tube, pleural tap), consider ordering a stat portable chest x-ray to check for pneumothorax or mediastinal widening (as seen occasionally in aortic aneurysm).

Inform RN

"Will arrive in . . . minutes."

Get to the patient as quickly as possible! Try to have the ECG started or at least set up for your arrival; it will save valuable time in the event of a true medical emergency. Remember that complaints of chest pain need to be evaluated without delay. Although patients on psychiatric wards typically are more stable medically, some also have co-morbid medical illnesses that might not be focused on as closely as on a medical floor.

■ ELEVATOR THOUGHTS

What can cause chest pain?
1. **Cardiac factors**
   a. Angina
   b. MI
   c. Aortic dissection
   d. Pericarditis
2. **Pulmonary factors**
   a. Pulmonary embolism
   b. Pneumothorax
   c. Pneumonia with pleuritis

3. **Gastrointestinal factors**
   a. Esophageal reflux or spasm, esophagitis
   b. Peptic ulcer disease
   c. Cholecystitis
4. **Musculoskeletal factors**
   a. Costal chondritis
   b. Rib fracture
   c. Muscle spasm
5. **Skin factors**
   a. Herpes zoster
6. **Psychiatric factors**
   a. Anxiety disorders
   b. Somatoform disorders
   c. Factitious disorder
   d. Substance-related disorders (e.g., amphetamine or cocaine intoxication/withdrawal)

■ MAJOR THREAT TO LIFE

- MI or myocardial ischemia
- Aortic dissection
- Pulmonary embolus
- Pneumothorax

Each of these situations represents a major threat to life and needs to be managed quickly. Generally, psychiatric wards are not adequately equipped to manage or monitor medical emergencies. **Do not try to be a hero.** You may feel confident in your abilities to manage medical issues, but these situations can get out of hand quickly and should be managed by those with more experience and who will be caring for the patient should he or she need to be transferred off the psychiatric ward.

If the situation appears likely to be one of those listed, get the medical consultant, cardiology consultant, or cardiac care unit (CCU) team involved right away. They will usually appreciate being involved early in the management and can be very helpful in facilitating transfer to the appropriate setting. Always evaluate the patient personally before calling the consultants. You will be better able to report the details of the situation that they will probably want to know.

■ BEDSIDE

Quick Look Test

Does the patient look well (comfortable), sick (uncomfortable or distressed), or critical (about to die?)

Where the art of medicine cannot be underestimated is in the quick look test. Overall appearance of the patient can usually provide important clues to the severity of a problem. Calm, conversant, and relatively comfortable-appearing patients are less likely to have a life-threatening cause of their chest pain. Patients with chest pain due to myocardial ischemia or MI usually appear pale, anxious, and diaphoretic. Keep in mind that although often accurate, this is a quick gauge of severity, and things are not always as they seem. A patient in the midst of a panic attack can appear just as ill as one suffering from an acute infarction. A patient with autonomic sensory neuropathy—for example, someone with advanced diabetes—might report vague or, indeed, even no pain during a severe MI. There is no substitute for getting a thorough history from the patient as well as an ECG.

Airway and Vital Signs

What is the patient's blood pressure?

Most patients who complain of chest pain will be normotensive. Hypotension can occur with MI, cardiogenic shock, pulmonary embolism, and tension pneumothorax. Hypertension may occur in the anxious patient with chest pain as well as in the patient with cocaine/amphetamine intoxication. Severe hypertension (systolic blood pressure [BP] > 180 mm Hg, diastolic BP > 110 mm Hg) should be treated, as it can worsen myocardial ischemia and aortic dissection.

What is the patient's heart rate?

Sinus tachycardia can occur with chest pain of any origin. If the heart rate is greater than 100 beats per minute, life-endangering tachydysrhythmias, such as ventricular tachycardia or atrial fibrillation, should be considered as medical emergencies. Immediate intervention, such as cardioversion, may be required.

Does the patient have bradycardia?

Although bradycardia can indicate myocardial ischemia or MI, in particular an inferior wall MI, unless it is dangerously slow it often may not require immediate treatment but should be monitored closely.

What is the patient's breathing pattern and quality?

A rapid respiratory rate can occur with any type of chest pain. It is important to remember that tachypnea may be a result of hypoxemia, which may result from myocardial ischemia or MI. Tachypnea also commonly accompanies panic attacks.

Painful breathing (dyspnea) most often indicates a pleural or musculoskeletal cause (pleuritis, pneumothorax, costal chondritis, rib fracture).

Mental Status Examination

Does the patient have signs of depression or anxiety?

You should perform an abbreviated mental status examination to identify conditions that should be treated urgently. A patient with somatic complaints may be very depressed and may even require a one-to-one observation. A patient having a panic attack will probably respond to a fast-acting benzodiazepine. A depressed patient with somatic complaints may often describe a depressed mood, have a constricted range of affect, and admit to suicidal ideation. An anxious patient may appear extremely agitated and frightened.

Selective History and Chart Review

One useful mnemonic for exploring the causes of chest pain is "PQRST":

P—What is the **P**osition/location of the pain?

Q—What is the **Q**uality of the pain (sharp, dull, ripping, tearing, pressure, squeezing, other)?

R—Does the pain **R**adiate to other locations (left arm, jaw, back, other)?

S—How does the patient rate the **S**everity of the pain (on a scale of 1 to 10)?

T—What is the **T**ime course of the pain (sudden onset, intermittent, constant, other)?

1. How does the patient describe the quality of the pain? Has the patient experienced the same kind of pain before?

    Crushing, squeezing, viselike pain or pressure is how MI is typically described. Severe tearing or ripping pain may indicate aortic dissection or peptic ulcer disease. Often patients who have had prior cardiac incidents will be able to tell you what they felt during their last episode.

2. Does the pain radiate?

    Radiation to the back may indicate peptic ulcer disease or aortic dissection. Myocardial infarction typically radiates to the jaw, neck, and left arm. Localized pain is often seen with rib fracture, costal chondritis, or trauma. A dermatomic distribution is classic for herpes zoster. Diffuse pain is nonspecific and could be an indication of somatization disorder or panic.

3. Does the pain change with deep breathing or coughing?

    Pain that changes may be pleuritic and suggests pleuritis,

fracture, costal chondritis, pneumonia, pericarditis, pulmonary embolism, or pneumothorax.

Selective Physical Examination

1. Vital signs
   a. Repeat
2. Respiratory
   a. Crackles (pneumonia; congestive heart failure [CHF], which may be secondary to MI; pulmonary embolism)
   b. Decreased breath sounds (consolidation, pleural effusion)
   c. Absence of breath sounds (pneumothorax)
3. Cardiovascular
   a. Murmurs, gallops, rubs (MI, pericarditis, CHF)
   b. Jugular venous distension (tension pneumothorax, CHF with right-sided heart failure, pulmonary embolus with right-sided strain/overload, pericardial effusion)
4. Abdominal
   a. Tenderness, guarding, or rebound (peptic ulcer disease with or without perforation)
5. Skin
   a. Rash in dermatomic distribution (herpes zoster)
6. Musculoskeletal
   a. Tenderness on palpation (costal chondritis, rib fracture, trauma)

■ MANAGEMENT

1. **Suspected myocardial ischemia or infarction:** The patient should be given **325 mg aspirin to chew** and **sublingual nitroglycerin 0.4 mg separated by 5 minutes up to three times,** making sure not to cause a drop in systolic BP below 90 mm Hg. Call the medical consultant, cardiology consultant, or CCU team right away to get them involved early so that the patient can be transferred to and managed in the appropriate setting. You are responsible for the care of the patient until the transfer of care is complete. You should attempt to stabilize the patient and start the appropriate medical work-up while awaiting transfer or arrival of the medical team.
2. **Stabilizing the patient for transfer should include**
   a. Monitoring vital signs
   b. Performing serial ECGs
   c. Obtaining routine laboratory tests (complete blood count [CBC], blood chemistries and creatine kinase with MB fraction, prothrombin and partial thromboplastin times)
   d. Getting a chest x-ray

e. Gaining intravenous access with the largest-gauge needle possible
f. Starting oxygen at 2 to 4 L/min or as recommended by the medical consult

3. **Pulmonary embolism:** Include portable chest x-ray and measure arterial blood gas while awaiting transfer to medicine.

4. **Pneumonia:** Include portable chest x-ray and send sputum for culture and sensitivity tests. If the patient is in respiratory distress, administer oxygen after getting recommendations on rate of delivery from the medical consult.

5. **Esophagitis:** If you feel confident that esophagitis is the correct diagnosis, the patient can be managed on the psychiatric unit without urgent medical attention and may be treated with an antacid such as aluminum hydroxide **(Maalox or Mylanta). 30 mL orally [PO] every 4 to 6 hours.** Elevation of the head may be helpful. Suggest a gastrointestinal (GI) consultation for the next day. Perform an ECG. It will not harm the patient and may show unexpected results.

6. **Peptic ulcer disease:** Antacids may be given, but they might not offer the patient much relief. Suggest a GI consultation for the next day.

7. **Costal chondritis:** Costal chondritis can be treated with non-steroidal anti-inflammatory drugs (NSAIDs) such as **ibuprofen 600 mg PO every 6 to 8 hours,** if not contraindicated secondary to other medical conditions (e.g., in a patient who is taking an anticoagulant or has peptic ulcer disease)

8. **Herpes zoster:** Initially the patient with herpes zoster may require pain treatment with NSAIDs or even narcotics, if not contraindicated. Suggest an infectious disease consult for the next day.

9. **Psychiatric:** The first course of action for any suspected psychiatric etiology is always a thorough psychiatric interview. Simple reassurance and support is frequently helpful for patients with panic attack, somatization disorders, or depression. If the patient remains anxious, treatment with a fast-acting benzodiazepine such as **lorazepam (Ativan) 1 to 2 mg PO or intramuscularly** can be initiated. It may be **repeated every 2 hours with a maximum dose of 10 mg in 24 hours.**

10. **Cocaine or amphetamine intoxication:** The patient with chest pain secondary to substance intoxication could be experiencing myocardial ischemia or even MI. Cocaine and amphetamines can cause life-threatening arrythmias, and an urgent medical consultation is indicated. Proceed with cardiac workup and management.

22 | Nausea and Vomiting

MADELEINE CASTELLANOS

■ BACKGROUND

Nausea is a subjective symptom of gastric discomfort, associated with the desire to vomit. It can result from a variety of sources, such as primary gastrointestinal (GI) disease, central nervous system (CNS) disorders, endocrine and metabolic disorders, systemic illness, and disorders of the thorax, or may be a side effect of certain medications (theophylline, digoxin, valproic acid, selective serotonin reuptake inhibitors [SSRIs], opiates, dopamine agonists). Pregnancy should always be ruled out in premenopausal women.

The act of vomiting occurs as the result of stimulation of two centers in the brain. The first is the vomiting center in the lateral reticular formation and is stimulated by efferent impulses that arise in the GI tract and elsewhere, such as in the heart and mesentery.

The second center is the chemoreceptor trigger zone in the floor of the fourth ventricle and is stimulated by many drugs and by metabolic abnormalities such as acidosis and uremia. The efferent impulses arise only in the vomiting center, and stimulation of the chemoreceptor trigger zone leads in turn to stimulation of the vomiting center.

Vomiting is usually preceded by nausea. Nausea is associated with a reduced gastric tone and an increased duodenal tone. Retching, which represents deep inspiratory movements against a closed glottis, follows the sensation of nausea. The final act of vomiting results from the sustained contractions of the muscles of the abdominal wall. It is important to distinguish between vomiting, which is the return of gastric and at times duodenal contents, and regurgitation, which is a symptom of esophageal disease. Regurgitation is unaccompanied by nausea, retching, or straining.

Vomiting is usually associated with a number of other phenomena. Tachycardia is common. Hypersalivation and diarrhea may also occur. (The control centers in the medulla for these phenomena are near the vomiting center.)

Certain characteristics of vomiting—its amount, duration, nature (content), and relationship to meals—are helpful in suggesting its cause. Vomiting of psychogenic origin (as in anorexia nervosa, bulimia, or certain psychotic or delusional states) occurs often just after or during meals and is characteristic in that the patient always manages to avoid vomiting in a public place. Early morning vomiting is a feature of anxiety states but can also occur in pregnancy, alcoholism, and uremia. Intestinal obstruction induces copious vomiting with bile present; the vomitus may also have a fecal odor. Vomiting of undigested food eaten several hours up to a day earlier suggests delayed gastric emptying. This could be the result of gastric outlet obstruction or motor disturbance of the stomach, such as that which occurs in diabetes, scleroderma, or hypokalemia.

The nature of the vomitus can provide information about the cause. In obstructive vomiting, the presence of bile indicates that obstruction is distal to the pylorus. Blood in the vomitus occurs only in esophageal, gastric, or duodenal disease and may represent an inflammatory or malignant process. In patients with alcohol abuse or dependence, bleeding from esophageal varices should be considered the cause of bloody vomitus until it can be ruled out by endoscopy. Prolonged vomiting of any cause may produce a tear in the lower esophageal or gastric fundal mucosa, which may bleed profusely (Mallory-Weiss syndrome).

The major categories of disorders associated with vomiting are
- Psychogenic
- Drug induced
- Intra-abdominal colic or sepsis
- Toxic or metabolic disorders
- Postsurgical vomiting
- Gastric outlet obstruction
- Intestinal obstruction
- Neurologic (intracranial) diseases
- Ingested poisons or toxins
- Viral gastroenteritis
- Cyclic vomiting of childhood
- Pregnancy
- Emotion or anxiety

Of these clinical entities, intra-abdominal, intracranial, and metabolic disorders demand immediate attention.

■ PHONE CALL

Questions

1. When did nausea and vomiting start?
2. What is the nature of the emesis (e.g., bright red blood, darker blood with clots, "coffee grounds," bilious, feculent odor, undigested food)?
3. What is the amount of the emesis (rough estimate of emesis volume and frequency)?
4. What are the associated vital signs (fever, tachycardia, hypotension)?

5. What are the associated signs and symptoms (abdominal, chest, back, pelvic, or rectal pain; diarrhea, constipation, relation to nausea)?
6. What are the patient's diagnoses and co-morbid conditions (history of abdominal or pelvic surgery, cardiac disease)?
7. Which medications is the patient taking? (Many medications can produce nausea, which may precede the vomiting.)
8. When was the patient admitted?
9. Is there any history of substance abuse?
10. How does the patient look now (nurse's estimate of how the patient is doing, e.g., moribund, distressed, resting quietly)?

Orders

If the patient is hypotensive, have an intravenous (IV) unit set up with a large-bore short catheter ready for insertion and give a **500-mL bolus of lactated Ringer's solution.**

If the emesis is bloody or in large amounts, order a Salem sump tube No. 18, an intermittent suction device (such as a Gomco machine), and an irrigation set to the bedside. Tell the nurse to save the vomitus for your inspection.

Inform RN

"Will arrive in . . . minutes."

Significant alterations in vital signs, pain, or significant amounts of bright red blood will require you to see the patient as soon as possible.

■ ELEVATOR THOUGHTS

Is the patient vomiting? If so, how much?

Did nausea precede the vomiting?

What are the causes of vomiting?
- GI disease
- CNS disorders
- Endocrine and metabolic disorders
- Systemic illness
- Disorders of the thorax
- Side effect of medications

What is the content of the vomitus? Does it contain blood?

What is the association with eating?

Is the patient pregnant?

Is there blood in the vomitus?

■ MANAGEMENT

Major threats to life with regard to intra-abdominal processes that may present with vomiting include the following:

- Gastric outlet obstruction
- Intestinal obstruction
- Gastrointestinal inflammation
- Perforation of a viscus
- Peritonitis
- Pancreatitis
- Intra-abdominal or pelvic abscess
- Acute distension of smooth muscle in the bile duct, ureter, or small intestine

Almost all of these disorders will present with nausea, vomiting, and associated signs and symptoms. The more ominous ones are a lack of bowel sounds, abdominal distension, tenderness, and guarding and rebound (the peritoneal signs), all of which indicate that a surgical consultation should be obtained in a timely manner.

Intracranial processes that may be associated with vomiting include those that lead to increased intracranial pressure (tumor, hematoma), migraine headaches, infection, gastric neuropathies, and many toxic and metabolic encephalopathies. Any change in the neurologic status requires the neurologist to evaluate the patient.

In most instances, however, nausea and vomiting are drug induced. In psychiatric patients, nausea and vomiting may be the result of pharmacotherapy or toxicity. For example, lithium toxicity and SSRI pharmacotherapy (as well as therapy with other psychotropic drugs) can cause nausea and vomiting. Anticholinergic agents may cause vomiting by inhibiting motor activity and causing partial gastric outlet obstruction. Therefore, this should be considered for patients taking these agents.

For any patient who has prolonged or severe vomiting, the initial management should include IV hydration; intermittent nasogastric suction; determination of baseline laboratory values, complete blood count, electrolytes, liver function tests, arterial blood gases, serum drug levels (for patients taking lithium, valproic acid, or digoxin), glucose, and lactate; and initiation of a search for etiology. These management protocols are outside the scope of psychiatry and require the appropriate medical, surgical, or neurologic consultation.

A note of caution regarding the pharmacotherapy of vomiting is warranted. The use of antiemetic or antinausea agents, such as hydroxyzine or prochlorperazine, should be avoided until the etiology of the vomiting is determined. As with all abdominal processes, pain should not be treated with narcotics or nonsteroidal anti-inflammatory drugs, as it is an important marker of the progression of many serious intra-abdominal processes, and the physician follows the nature of this pain as an important aid in diagnosis.

MARKUS J. KRAEBBER

Extreme changes in body temperature in psychiatric inpatients should be a cause for concern. Depending on the working diagnosis and initial treatment, fever can be an early sign of an impending disease process, with accompanying morbidity and mortality. Even temperature elevations that are not extreme, including those to about 100.5°F, warrant timely evaluation. **If a fever work-up is negative and the patient is on an antipsychotic medication, think about neuroleptic malignant syndrome (NMS).**

■ **PHONE CALL**

Questions

1. What is the temperature, and how was it taken (e.g., orally or rectally)?
2. What time was the temperature taken?
3. What are the other vital signs?
4. What are the associated symptoms and signs (if any)?
5. What has been the trend in the patient's temperature over the past 24 to 48 hours?
6. What is the admission diagnosis?
7. What was the date of admission?
8. What co-morbid medical or surgical conditions exist in this patient? Have there been any recent medical or surgical procedures (e.g., blood transfusion or bronchoscopy)?
9. What is the patient's substance use history?
10. Is the patient taking an antipsychotic? If so, for how long?
11. Has the patient's intake or output changed in any way?
12. How does the patient look (nurse's estimate of the patient's condition)?

Orders

1. If other vital signs were not taken, have them taken now.
2. If the patient is hypotensive with fever, order an intravenous

setup and have a **fluid bolus of 500 mL of lactated Ringer's or normal saline solution** given. If the patient is hemodynamically unstable, get the medical consultant involved immediately.
3. If the patient has symptoms and signs of meningitis (nuchal rigidity, mental status changes, photophobia), order a lumbar puncture tray to the ward.
4. Have the nurse order blood culture trays and obtain a urinalysis (U/A) with culture and sensitivity (C&S).

Inform RN

"Will arrive in . . . minutes."
The possibility of septic shock, meningitis, pulmonary embolism, delirium tremens, barbiturate withdrawal, or NMS demands that you see the patient immediately.

■ ELEVATOR THOUGHTS

What are causes of fever and change in temperature in psychiatric patients?
1. Infection: bacterial, viral, parasitic, fungal (e.g., urinary tract infection [UTI] in an elderly patient, right upper or middle lobe pneumonia in a patient with a history of alcohol abuse, aspiration of excess saliva from clozapine therapy, an infectious agent in an immunocompromised patient, or infection or abscess in a patient who has had a recent surgical or dental procedure)
2. Drug-induced fever (e.g., NMS, medication side effect)—**is the patient on an antipsychotic medication?**
3. Pulmonary embolism (PE)
4. Deep vein thrombosis (DVT)
5. Substance withdrawal
6. Neoplastic syndromes
7. Autoimmune or connective tissue disease
8. Postoperative/post-procedure fever (atelectasis, UTI, wound infections, DVT, PE)

■ MAJOR THREAT TO LIFE

- Septic shock
- Meningitis
- NMS
- Alcohol-related delirium tremens
- Withdrawal
- PE

■ BEDSIDE

Quick Look Test

Is the patient resting comfortably, sick, distressed, agitated, apprehensive, lethargic, stuporous, catatonic, or comatose?

Airway, Breathing, Circulation, and Vital Signs

1. **Airway:** Can the patient maintain his or her airway? Are accessory muscles of respiration in use? Is there stridor?
2. **Breathing:** What are the respiratory rate and quality? Is there evidence of hypoxia (e.g., cyanosis, increased respiratory rate)? If you have evidence of cardiopulmonary arrest or suspect that one is imminent, have the nurse call a cardiac arrest code and get the arrest cart to the bedside. Initiate advanced cardiac life support (ACLS) protocols.
3. **Pulse rate:** Often the febrile patient is tachycardic; expect a rise in the pulse rate of 10 beats per minute with each degree Fahrenheit (or 16 beats for each degree Celsius) increase in temperature.

   Bradycardia in the febrile patient has been associated with falciparum malaria with profound hemolysis, typhoid fever, both *Mycoplasma* pneumonia and *Legionella* pneumonia, and ascending cholangitis.
4. **Blood pressure:** Hypotension and fever (or a decrease in body temperature) can be indicative of septic shock. Assess the patient's volume status and initiate intravenous (IV) fluid challenge **(500 mL of lactated Ringer's or normal saline solution)** via a large-bore peripheral IV catheter. Call for a medical consult as this probably warrants transfer to a medical ward.
5. **Circulation:** In addition to assessing the pulse rate and blood pressure, one can determine circulatory status by assessing the skin color, capillary refill, and sensorium.

   There are two stages in the development of septic shock. Warm shock occurs first. Increased cardiac output and peripheral vasodilation cause the skin to be warm, dry, and flushed. The second stage is the development of cold shock, in which the patient becomes hypotensive and peripheral vasoconstriction occurs, leaving the skin cool and clammy. Changes in sensorium ranging from lethargy to agitation can occur with fever, particularly in the elderly. If a specific cause for fever is not obvious, a lumbar puncture (LP) should be performed to rule out meningitis.

Selective Physical Examination I

Keep in mind volume status, signs and symptoms of septic shock, and signs and symptoms of meningitis.

1. **Vital signs:** Repeat. Check skin for turgor, temperature, color, and moistness.
2. **Head, eyes, ears, nose, and throat (HEENT):** Evaluate the tongue, oral mucous membranes, and conjunctivae for moistness. Look for photophobia and neck stiffness. Assess the jugular venous pulse waves.
3. **Respiratory function:** Note the rate and quality. Is there any respiratory distress? Assess lung fields for crackles, wheezes, or decreased breath sounds.
4. **Cardiac function:** Note the pulse rate. Assess the pulse volume, and check the distal capillary refill.
5. **Abdomen:** Note any tenderness.
6. **Neurologic:** Assess for acute changes in mental status (agitation, lethargy, catatonia). Look for rigidity associated with NMS. Look for signs of the autonomic hyperactivity associated with substance withdrawal (increase in pulse rate, blood pressure, and temperature, as well as sweating, tremors, piloerection, and tongue fasciculations) and for signs of autonomic instability associated with NMS.
7. **Special maneuvers:** Assess the patient for Brudzinski's sign and Kernig's sign (each is suggestive of meningeal irritation).

Management I

Major life-threatening situations include the following:
1. **Septic shock:** Volume-resuscitate aggressively (use caution with patients who have a history of heart failure). While resuscitation is in progress, measure prothrombin and partial thromboplastin times, fibrinogen, fibrin split products, electrolytes, blood urea nitrogen, creatinine, glucose, serum alanine transaminase (ALT), serum aspartate transaminase (AST), gamma-glutamyltransferase (GGT), alkaline phosphatase, amylase, total and direct bilirubin, lactate dehydrogenase (LDH), and creatine kinase (important for shock status). Order a complete blood count with differential count (T-cell profiles in immunocompromised patients). Obtain aerobic and anaerobic blood culture specimens from two separate sites. Obtain urine for U/A with microscopic U/A and urine for Gram's stain and culture. Obtain sputum for Gram's stain and culture, including tests for acid-fast bacilli (AFB). Measure arterial blood gas to determine the base deficit (the greater the deficit, the more profound or prolonged the shock).

A patient in septic shock will most likely be transferred to a medical intensive care unit (ICU) or a surgical ICU if this has occurred after a surgical procedure. The patient will need broad-spectrum antibiotics and will require intensive monitoring. Other ICU supportive measures may be needed, including intubation and ventilatory support.

2. **Meningitis:** Perform an ophthalmic examination to rule out papilledema (increased intracranial pressure) and a complete neurologic examination. If meningitis is suspected, a neurologic consultation should be requested. An LP, with measurement of cerebrospinal fluid (CSF) pressures and collection of CSF for appropriate studies and cultures, should be performed as quickly as possible. In some instances, a computed tomography (CT) scan of the head may be necessary before LP to help rule out increased intracranial pressure and possible herniation. Ideally, IV antibiotics are begun immediately after the LP and collection of CSF specimens for studies. If the patient requires a head CT before the LP, however, do not wait to begin the IV antibiotics. In addition, blood cultures and laboratory tests, as outlined for septic shock, should be obtained. Fever, headache, seizure, stiff neck, or changes in sensorium should be considered evidence of meningitis until proven otherwise. The appropriate neurologic or medical consultant should be contacted to evaluate the patient. Collection of CSF should be done as rapidly as possible unless the patient has a coagulopathy, papilledema is present, or focal neurologic signs exist, which are highly suspicious for the presence of a mass lesion. Inform the consultant of these facts. You may elect to begin IV antibiotics empirically and obtain an immediate noncontrast head CT (if available) to rule out any space-occupying lesions.

3. **Pulmonary embolism:** Depending on the size and location of the embolus, the patient's outcome can range from immediate death to a mild cough with fever. You should have a suspicion of PE for patients who are restrained for prolonged periods of time, are bedridden for medical or surgical reasons, or have a history of DVT or hypercoagulable states. Localizing signs and symptoms include shortness of breath, cough, chest pain, hemoptysis, crackles or a friction rub on auscultation, dullness to percussion, egophony and bronchophony, whispered pectoriloquy, Westermark's sign on chest x-ray, and characteristic changes on electrocardiogram. A medical consultation should be called, as the patient will probably require anticoagulation medication (unless contraindications exist) and further radiologic tests.

4. **Delirium tremens:** See Chapter 18.

5. **Barbiturate withdrawal:** See Chapter 18.

6. **Neuroleptic malignant syndrome:** See Chapter 14. **This clinical entity should be high on the list of possibilities in the differential diagnosis for any patient on an antipsychotic medication.** Obtain blood work for creatine kinase levels.

Selective Chart Review

If the patient does not have one of the previously discussed causes for fever, do a selective chart review, looking for localizing clues from the following:

- Admission history and physical examination
- Process of medical clearance to psychiatry (e.g., what was done, what was recommended, what is pending, consultations, tests)
- Current medications (steroids, antipyretics, antibiotics, antipsychotics)
- Allergies
- Substance use history (when the patient last used a substance)
- Recent laboratory values
- Temperature trends during hospitalization
- Evidence of immunodeficiency (e.g., human immunodeficiency virus [HIV] infection, acquired immunodeficiency syndrome [AIDS], cancer chemotherapy, malignancy)
- Other reasons for fever (autoimmune disease, neoplasm, drug fever, substance withdrawal)

Selective Physical Examination II

Search to confirm localizing symptoms and signs that may exist as suggested by the chart review.

1. **Vital signs:** repeat now (rectal temperature, if possible)
2. **HEENT:**
   - **Fundi:** papilledema (intracranial abscess), Roth's spots (infective endocarditis)
   - **Conjunctiva:** scleral petechiae (infective endocarditis)
   - **Ears:** erythematous tympanic membrane (otitis media)
   - **Sinuses:** tenderness, inability to transilluminate (sinusitis)
   - **Oral cavity:** dental caries and abscess
   - **Pharynx:** erythema, exudate (pharyngitis, thrush, tonsillar abscess)
   - **Neck:** meningeal signs, lymphadenopathy
3. **Chest:** crackles, friction rub, egophony, bronchophony, other signs of consolidation (pneumonia, pulmonary embolism)
4. **Cor:** new murmurs (infective endocarditis), pericardial friction rub (pericarditis)
5. **Abdomen and back:** localized tenderness, guarding, rebound costovertebral angle tenderness (pyelonephritis)
6. **Rectal:** tenderness or mass (perirectal abscess)
7. **Pelvic:** tenderness or mass (pelvic inflammatory disease, cervicitis)
8. **Extremities:** calf swelling and tenderness, Homans' sign

(DVT), joint tenderness, swelling, erythema, effusion (septic joint)
9. **Skin:** examine, including IV sites, for possible tenderness or rashes. Look for rubor, dolor, calor, tumor, pressure sores (infection and abscess), petechiae (infective endocarditis), Osler's nodes, Janeway lesions (any surgical wound must be exposed and examined)

Management II

Any patient with an unexplained rectal temperature of 38°C or greater needs the following:

1. Aerobic and anaerobic blood cultures from two separate sites
2. U/A (with microscopy) and urine culture
3. White blood count and differential
4. Other more selective tests, depending on localizing clues elicited from your chart review, history, and physical examination, such as
   a. Throat swabs for Gram's stain and culture
   b. Sputum for Gram's stain, AFB stain, and cultures
   c. Chest x-ray
   d. LP
   e. Special-protocol blood cultures (e.g., AFB, fungal)
   f. Swabs for Gram's stain and aerobic and anaerobic cultures from all sites that appear infected or are drawing fluid
   g. Studies for parasites and other infectious agents
   h. Obtain blood work for creatine kinase determination to rule out NMS (if the patient is on an antipsychotic medication)

Once the data acquisition and initial fever work-up have begun, appropriate consultation with the medical, neurologic, or surgical services should be obtained to determine the appropriate antibiotic therapy and management of the patient.

Keep in mind which patient will need broad-spectrum antibiotics immediately:

1. The patient with fever and hypotension
2. The patient with fever and neutropenia ($<1000/mm^3$) or other signs and symptoms or history of immunocompromise
3. The patient who is febrile and appears acutely ill or toxic

The following types of patients need specific antibiotics immediately:

1. The patient with fever and meningeal signs and symptoms
2. The patient with fever and clear localizing signs and symptoms

Remember, with any serious change in the status of a patient, inform the patient's attending physician and never hesitate to ask for help from the appropriate attending or consulting service.

Once again, for any patient taking antipsychotic medication who has a fever, you must fully consider NMS (see Chapter 14).

24 | Seizures

Erwin C. Ting

Seizure is a generic term for an episode of abnormal neurologic function secondary to abnormal electrical discharge of neurons. The epilepsies constitute a group of disorders characterized by chronic, recurrent, paroxysmal changes in neurologic function secondary to abnormal electrical activity of neurons. The physician on call must manage the seizure and give an accurate account of the observed phenomena to the primary clinician or neurologic consultant.

■ PHONE CALL

Questions

1. Has the seizure stopped? Is the patient conscious?
2. Did someone witness the seizure? If so, ask for a specific description.
3. What are the patient's vital signs? Does the patient have a fever? Is the blood pressure elevated?
4. What are the patient's age, sex, diagnosis, and medications?
5. If the patient is female, is she pregnant?
6. Does the patient have a history of seizures?
7. Are there any obvious injuries?

Orders

1. Move the patient into the lateral decubitus position to avoid aspiration. Take special care with head and neck injuries.
2. Have available
   - Airway setup
   - Intravenous setup
   - Apparatus for blood collection
3. If the patient is postictal, remove any dentures and suction the oropharynx.
4. Ask for a Chemstrip reading for glucose.
5. Ask someone to stay with the patient.
6. Advise nursing personnel to avoid active restraint because perceived threat can result in defensive reactions dangerous to the caregiver.

Inform RN

"Will arrive in . . . minutes."

Note: A patient who is experiencing a seizure must be seen immediately.

■ ELEVATOR THOUGHTS

Was the attack truly a seizure?

Any paroxysmal event that transiently alters neurologic function can be mistaken for an epileptic seizure. The differential diagnosis includes the following:

1. **Cardiac arrhythmias, vasovagal syncope, and postural hypotension** can produce loss of consciousness and result in brief generalized clonic movements if cerebral hypoxia is prolonged.

2. **Complicated migraine** can mimic focal sensory seizures or present as an acute confusional state resembling an absence seizure or complex partial status epilepticus.

3. **Transient ischemic attacks** may be manifested as brief, repetitive, stereotyped sensory or motor deficits, amnesia, or aphasia.

4. **Transient global amnesia** can produce sudden confusion and acute loss of memory. Cognitive functions and language remain intact, and these attacks occur rarely.

5. **Sleep disorders** include narcolepsy, cataplexy (may mimic an atonic seizure), and parasomnias (sleepwalking, night terrors).

6. **Movement disorders** include tics, Tourette's syndrome, myoclonus, and choreoathetosis.

7. **Nonepileptic psychogenic seizure (hysterical seizures or pseudoseizures)** are suggested by bizarre facial grimacing, body posturing, opisthotonus, pelvic thrusting, and completely asynchronous thrashing of limbs. This type of seizure is most common in patients with a history of sexual, physical, or substance abuse; personality disorder; or other psychiatric illness. Patients may also have a real seizure disorder, and video electroencephalogram (EEG) monitoring may be required to make the diagnosis.

What kind of seizure was it?

1. **Partial (focal and local) seizures**
   a. Simple partial seizures (consciousness not impaired)
      (1) With motor symptoms
      (2) With somatosensory or special sensory symptoms (simple hallucinations, tingling, light flashing, buzzing)
      (3) With autonomic symptoms or signs (e.g., epigastric sensation, pallor, sweating, flushing, piloerection, pupillary dilation)

   (4) With psychic symptoms (disturbances of higher cerebral function—e.g., déjà vu, fear, distortion of time perception)

  b. Complex partial seizures (impairment of consciousness and often automatisms)

   (1) With simple partial onset followed by impairment of consciousness

   (2) With impairment of consciousness at onset

  c. Partial seizures evolving to secondary generalized seizures (e.g., generalized tonic-clonic seizures)

   (1) Simple partial seizures evolving to generalized seizures

   (2) Complex partial seizures evolving to generalized seizures

   (3) Simple partial seizures evolving to complex partial seizures and further evolving to generalized seizures

2. Generalized seizures (convulsive or nonconvulsive)

  a. Absence seizures (petit mal): impairment of consciousness alone or with mild clonic, atonic, or tonic components and automatisms

  b. Tonic, clonic, tonic-clonic (grand mal)

  c. Myoclonic

  d. Atonic

  e. Infantile spasms

  f. Atypical absence

3. Status epilepticus

  a. Tonic-clonic status

  b. Absence status

  c. Epilepsia partialis continua

What caused the seizure?

1. Infection

  a. Meningitis

  b. Encephalitis

  c. Abscess

  d. Granuloma

2. Neoplasm

  a. Primary

  b. Metastatic

3. Vascular

  a. Ischemic, hemorrhagic stroke

  b. Vasculitis

  c. Arteriovenous malformation

  d. Hypertensive encephalopathy

4. Metabolic

  a. Hypoglycemia or hyperglycemia

  b. Hyponatremia (consider polydipsia)

  c. Hypocalcemia

  d. Hypoxia or hypercapnia

  e. Renal failure

5. **Head trauma**
   a. Acute
   b. History of trauma
6. **Drugs and toxins**
   a. Stopping antiepileptic medication or fall in therapeutic level
   b. Alcohol
   c. Benzodiazepine withdrawal, flumazenil
   d. Barbiturate withdrawal
   e. Lidocaine
   f. Antibiotics
      (1) Penicillins
      (2) Isoniazid (INH)
      (3) Cephalosporins
      (4) Ciprofloxacin
   g. Cyclic antidepressants
   h. Other antidepressants
      (1) Bupropion (Wellbutrin)
      (2) Maprotiline (Ludiomil)
      (3) Trazodone (Desyrel)
   i. Neuroleptics (especially clozapine)
   j. Lithium carbonate
   k. Drugs of abuse
      (1) Cocaine
      (2) Amphetamines
      (3) Lysergic acid diethylamide (LSD)
      (4) Marijuana
      (5) Phencyclidine hydrochloride (PCP)
      (6) Opioids (including meperidine)
   l. Hypoglycemics
   m. Anticholinergics
   n. Antihistamines
   o. Nonsteroidal anti-inflammatory drugs (NSAIDs)
   p. Sympathomimetics
   q. Carbon monoxide
7. **Hereditary disorders**
   a. Neurofibromatosis
   b. Sturge-Weber syndrome
   c. Tuberous sclerosis
8. **Febrile convulsions**
9. **Idiopathic**
10. **Nutritional**
    a. Pyridoxine deficiency
11. **Immunologic disorders**
    a. Systemic lupus erythematosus (SLE)
    b. Serum sickness

What are causes of seizures in older patients?
1. **Poststroke seizures and epilepsy**

   a. Occlusive vascular disease
   b. Intracranial hemorrhage
   c. Subarachnoid hemorrhage
   d. Post–carotid endarterectomy hyperperfusion syndrome
2. **Intracranial tumors**
3. **Degenerative disorders**
   a. Dementia
   b. Amyloid angiopathy
4. **Toxic metabolic disorders**
   a. Reflex epilepsy and nonketotic hyperglycemia in the elderly
   b. Seizure-associated speech arrest
   c. Seizures occurring after cardiac arrest
   d. Drug-induced seizures
5. **Undetermined**

   What evaluation is necessary?
   The flow chart presented in Figure 24–1 suggests some pertinent laboratory tests that should be considered.

■ MANAGEMENT

Principles of Seizure Management

   ▪ Stabilize the patient and attend to airway, breathing, and circulation.
   ▪ Obtain intravenous access, monitor vital signs, and arrange for routine and special laboratory tests.
   ▪ If the seizure does not stop within 5 to 10 minutes, treat as status epilepticus (usually with a combination of intravenous phenytoin and benzodiazepines as first-line therapy).
   ▪ Rule out intrinsic nervous system abnormality with clinical assessment, spinal fluid examination, neuroimaging, and special studies as indicated.
   ▪ Obtain reliable collateral history when available.
   ▪ Consider psychogenic or nonepileptic seizures.
   ▪ If nonconvulsive or subtle status epilepticus is likely, perform early EEG.
   ▪ Consider unusual presentation of systemic disorder (e.g., sarcoidosis, porphyria).
   ▪ Obtain drug history, and check all currently taken medications (including investigational drugs).
   ▪ Consider inadvertent or unrecognized drug or alcohol withdrawal.
   ▪ Consider illicit drug use, and obtain urine toxicology.
   ▪ Obtain history of possible environmental exposure to proconvulsant toxins.
   ▪ If the patient has a history of poorly controlled hypertension or if the blood pressure remains high 1 to 2 hours after seizure activity starts, consider hypertensive encephalopathy as the cause.

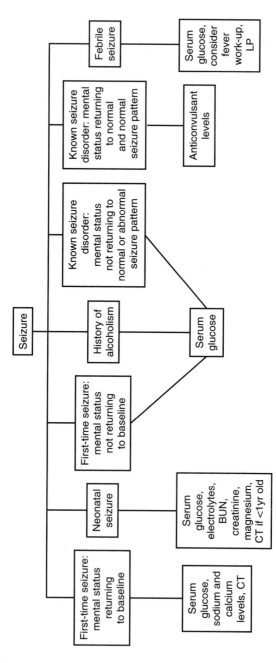

Figure 24–1 □ Flow chart showing pertinent laboratory tests for seizures. BUN = blood urea nitrogen; CT = computed tomography; LP = lumbar puncture.

- Correct all underlying potential causes as early as possible. Prescribe specific antidotes (e.g., intravenous pyridoxine for refractory alcohol-related seizures).

Status Epilepticus: A Medical Emergency

In status epilepticus (SE), seizures occur repeatedly, and cerebral function does not recover fully between seizures. It is also defined as continuous clinical or electrical seizure activity lasting more than 30 minutes whether or not consciousness is impaired. Noncompliance with anticonvulsant medication is an important cause of SE in epileptic patients. In patients without epilepsy, the causes of SE include alcohol withdrawal, acute intracerebral events such as stroke and intracerebral hemorrhage, central nervous system (CNS) infections, neoplasms, drug intoxication, anoxic encephalopathy, and acute metabolic disturbances. Abuse of cocaine, PCP, or amphetamine can also provoke SE.

Status epilepticus is a medical emergency that requires management in the intensive care unit with close monitoring. Time is critical because the morbidity and mortality rates increase with duration of seizure activity. Treatment includes the following:

- Stabilize the vital physiologic functions: Maintain airway, administer O_2, prevent aspiration, and maintain blood pressure.
- Draw blood to check glucose, electrolytes, calcium, and magnesium levels. Obtain a complete blood count and toxicology screens. Start an intravenous line and administer **100 mg of thiamine followed by 50 mL of 50% glucose**, and start intravenous antiepileptic medications.
- Start with **lorazepam in a dose of 0.1 mg/kg at 2 mg/min to a total dose of 8 mg**.
- If lorazepam fails to stop the SE, give **fosphenytoin in a loading dose of 20 mg/kg**. If SE persists, the initial dose may be followed by additional doses of **10 mg/kg** Hypotension frequently occurs in older patients. Therefore, it may be necessary to slow the rate of infusion or consider dopamine or other pressor agents.
- If SE persists, an endotracheal tube should be inserted for respiratory support and **phenobarbital (20 mg/kg) started at a rate of 50 to 100 mg/min**. For refractory SE, a pentobarbital coma may be required.

■ SEIZURE PRECAUTIONS

- Place bed in the lowest position
- Have oral airway at the head of the bed
- Put side rails (padded for tonic-clonic seizure) up when the patient is in bed

Table 24-1 □ TREATMENT WITH ANTIEPILEPTIC DRUGS ACCORDING TO
TYPE OF SEIZURE AND EPILEPTIC SYNDROME

Type of Seizure and Epileptic Syndrome	First-Line Drugs	Second-Line Drugs
Primary generalized seizures		
Absence seizures	Ethosuximide, valproic acid	Lamotrigine
Myoclonic seizures	Valproic acid	Acetazolamide, clonazepam, lamotrigine, primidone
Tonic-clonic seizures	Valproic acid, carbamazepine, phenytoin	Lamotrigine, phenobarbital, primidone
Juvenile myoclonic epilepsy	Valproic acid	Acetazolamide, clonazepam, primidone, lamotrigine
Infantile spasms	Corticotropin	Clonazepam, valproic acid
Partial seizures (all types)	Carbamazepine, phenytoin	Gabapentin, lamotrigine, phenobarbital, primidone, tiagabine topiramate, valproic acid

- Provide firm pillow
- Have suction at the bedside
- Have oxygen at the bedside
- Allow bathroom privileges with supervision only
- Allow bath or shower only with nurse in attendance
- Measure axilla temperature only
- Allow use of sharp objects (e.g., straight razor, nail scissors) with direct supervision only

There are three stages to the management of new-onset seizure:
1. Control continuing seizure activity
2. Treat any underlying disease
3. Prevent recurrent seizures

Long-term management of seizure disorders should be provided by a neurologist. A neurology consultation should always be obtained when dealing with new-onset seizures.

Tables 24–1 and 24–2 list medications and dosages appropriate for epileptic seizures.

Table 24-2 □ ANTIEPILEPTIC DRUGS AND DOSAGES

Medication	Adult Dose (mg/day)	Pediatric Dose (mg/kg/day)
Phenytoin	200–500	4–7
Carbamazepine	600–1600	5–20
Valproic acid	1000–3000	10–15
Phenobarbital	90–180	2–6
Primidone	300–1500	10–20
Ethosuximide	750–1500	15–40
Fosphenytoin	See below*	See below*
Gabapentin	900–4800	10–30
Lamotrigine	200–700	5–15
Topiramate	200–800	1–9
Vigabatrin	2000–4000	50–150
Tiagabine	32–56	0.25–1.5
Oxcarbazepine	1200–2400	—
Levetiracetam	1000–3000	—

*Loading dose in status epilepticus: 15–20 mg/kg intravenously (IV) at 150 mg/min in adults or 2–3 mg/kg/min in children weighing <50 kg; maintenance dose: 4–7 mg/kg intramuscularly or IV at 150 mg/min in adults or 2–3 mg/kg/min in children <50 kg twice daily.

25 | Falls

NOAH L. ROSEN
SIDDHARTHA NADKARNI

The physician on call is often asked to assess a patient who has fallen. All falls must be assessed rapidly and fully. In general, injury is the sixth leading cause of death after age 65 years, and about 5% to 10% of falls by the elderly lead to injury. The rate of falling is higher in long-term care facilities than at home, as patients frequently fall when trying to remove restraints, when going to the bathroom, and when trying to get out of bed in an unfamiliar place. Because of increased difficulty at night owing to less lighting, fewer people to assist with transfers, and confusion, those who are prone to fall include those who

- Are elderly
- Have a history of falling
- Have medical problems
- Have had recent or current intravenous or electro-convulsive therapy
- Have impaired gait
- Have poor vision or proprioception
- Are taking hypotensive or sedating medication
- Have dementia

■ PHONE CALL

Questions

1. Was the fall witnessed?
2. Is there an obvious injury?
3. What are the vital signs, including orthostatic changes?
4. Are there any acute changes in mental status or in level of arousal?
5. Is the patient receiving anticoagulants, antiepileptics, or sedating medication?
6. What were the medical and/or psychiatric diagnoses on admission?
7. Does the patient have a history of falling?
8. Does the patient have any localized pain, hematoma, or bleeding?

Orders

Ask the RN to notify you immediately if there are any changes (particularly in the mental status, level of arousal, or vital signs) before you are able to assess the patient. Give other appropriate orders as necessary (e.g., one-to-one observation, bed rest, frequent neurologic examinations).

Priorities

All falls must be evaluated as soon as possible. Definitively witnessed trivial falls may be tended to rapidly, but more severe falls may require comprehensive medical evaluation. Be aware that some falls may be described initially as minor, but you may find serious or rapidly progressive injury (e.g., head injury in a patient taking an antiplatelet or blood-thinning agent).

■ ELEVATOR THOUGHTS

Why does a patient fall?

Think primarily of environmental, cardiac, and neurologic causes. Your differential diagnosis should include

- Myocardial infarction (MI)
- Arrhythmias (particularly atrial fibrillation)
- Orthostasis (volume depletion, drugs, autonomic changes)
- Vasovagal reflex (notably in elderly patients going to the bathroom)
- Untended physical disabilities
- Confusion
- Delirium (especially in patients taking narcotics, sedatives, tricyclic antidepressants, tranquilizers, cimetidine, antihypertensives)
- Metabolic disorders
- Electrolyte abnormalities (think about Ca, Mg, Na, K)
- Hepatic and renal failure (may also increase exogenous drug levels)
- Dementia (Parkinson's disease and other subcortical processes, Alzheimer's disease, vascular disease, hydrocephalus/normal-pressure hydrocephalus)
- Transient ischemic attack (defined as occurring for a period less than 24 hours)
- Cerebrovascular accident
- Seizure (obtain a clear history as partial complex seizures are often overlooked)
- Environmental causes (e.g., disorientation at night [sundowning], a call bell that is not accessible, a wet floor, unassisted transfers out of bed, walking without assistance)

- Ataxia, including medication-induced ataxia (e.g., from carbamazepine)
- Multiple sensory deficits (e.g., poor vision, impaired proprioception)
- Diminished muscle strength
- Volitional falls (e.g., by psychotic, manic, or personality-disordered patients or by patients seeking primary or secondary gain)

■ MEDICAL AND NEUROLOGIC EMERGENCIES

A fall may be the result of an underlying medical emergency (e.g., MI, embolism). Even environmentally induced falls or slips can result in a serious injury that constitutes an emergency. Head injury usually warrants an immediate complete neurologic examination to rule out an intracranial bleed. Order a head computed tomography scan immediately if a new neurologic deficit is identified. For a patient taking anticoagulation medication, an immediate reversal of coagulation should be discussed with the medical or neurology consultant. Order frequent neurologic examinations and vital sign checks if no neurologic deficits are identified after a fall.

■ BEDSIDE

Quick Look Test

Does the patient look well, sick, or critical? Is there any evidence of injury or pain?

Airway and Vital Signs

What is the heart rate, and how is the rhythm?
Rule out arrhythmias.

Is the patient breathing normally?

What is the patient's level of arousal (awake, lethargic, obtunded, comatose)?

Orthostasis

Are orthostatic changes noted in heart rate (HR) or blood pressure (BP?)

Are there any drug-induced orthostatic changes?
Look at the actual medication dosing on the nurse's medication sheets.

Is there any evidence of volume depletion (BP and HR both change) or autonomic problems (BP drops but HR does not change)?

Selective History

Always obtain the full history from the patient, staff, any observers, and the chart. Remember that people's memories are often biased, and relevant facts must always be verified.

1. Was the fall witnessed?
2. Why did the patient fall?
3. Where did the patient fall?
4. What was the patient doing?
5. Were there any warning symptoms or signs of an impending fall?
6. Is there a history of previous falls? If so, were they similar?
7. Is there a history of hypoglycemia or diabetes?
8. Is there any injury or localizing pain?

Assess the patient's judgment and insight.

Selective Physical Examination

1. Vital signs (changes may indicate orthostatic hypotension, infection, arrhythmias)
2. Head, eyes, ears, nose, and throat (be sure to look for any sensory deficits, "raccoon eyes," cerebrospinal fluid loss, or significant bruising)
3. Cardiac (listen for arrhythmias, extra heart sounds, or rubs)
4. Musculoskeletal, especially pelvis (always have the patient fully rotate joints, as lack of movement may obscure a complete examination, and press on back, pelvis, and hips to check for pain on palpation)
5. Neurologic (including testing strength, reflexes, sensory, and especially gait)
6. Mental status examination (MSE) (especially orientation and cognition)

Selective Chart Review

1. Note the reasons for admission on Axis I, II, and III.
2. Look for a history of arrhythmia, seizures, autonomic dysfunction, nocturnal confusion, diabetes, dementia, multiple sensory deficits, or any other potentially causative medical diagnoses.
3. Review all current medications, including all available as-needed (PRN). Look especially for hypotensive agents, including cardiac medication, low-potency neuroleptics, tricyclic antidepressants, and other sedating medications.

4. Review the most recent laboratory tests and any changes (e.g., SMA 20, complete blood count [CBC] with differential count, acutely elevated liver function tests, elevated prothrombin and partial thromboplastin times and INR, drug levels, toxicology screens). Consider repeating laboratory tests that may be significant.

At this point, if you have any questions, contact the medical or neurologic consultant on call.

■ MANAGEMENT

Provisional Diagnosis

Establish the reason for the fall. A fall can be secondary to gait problems, balance problems, weakness, medication, and other medical conditions. Other causes include adverse drug reactions, syncopal episodes, new cerebrovascular accident (CVA), and onset of new medical condition. The reasons for a fall may often be multifactorial, and all contributing factors should be taken into account. For a patient with chronic risk factors, a slight change in treatment may substantially compromise activities of daily living.

Accidental falls frequently include rolling out of bed, tripping, or slipping. Always remember volitional falls in a psychiatric population with personality disorders and psychotic symptoms. If the suspicion of a volitional fall is raised, be sure to assess for the possibility of primary and secondary gain.

Complications

1. Fractures (hip fractures are the most common and carry a significant risk of morbidity and mortality)
2. Hemorrhage, hematoma (including those in nonobvious areas such as the thoracic cavity, the thigh, or the retroperitoneal space)
3. Lacerations
4. Other injuries

Call medical, neurologic, surgical, or orthopedic consultants immediately as appropriate.

■ TREAT THE CAUSE

As previously described, a fall may be a symptom of a medical or psychiatric illness or may be related to a side effect of medication. Identify and treat the illness (e.g., correct fluids and electrolytes, abort a seizure, hydrate), and discontinue or adjust the suspected medication. Plan for active prevention by providing assistance, supervision, surveillance, and appropriate teaching. Warn the patient and provide for safety precautions with a call bell, one-to-one observation, and adequate light. Keeping bed rails up may actually increase morbidity from falls; consider lowering the mattress to the floor. Correct all reversible factors, including treating occult urinary tract infections and nocturia, and address withdrawal from drugs or alcohol. Be aware that chronic alcoholic patients are prone to Wernicke's encephalopathy from acute thiamine depletion in the presence of a carbohydrate load (sugary meal).

Follow up with any consulting physicians already involved in the case. Take a proactive approach, and obtain pertinent laboratory results with CBC, therapeutic drug monitoring, prothrombin and partial thromboplastin times, SMA 20, chemical strips for glucose, urinalysis, and urine toxicology.

Finally, ensure that your full evaluation, consultants' notes, tests obtained, and actions taken are fully documented in the chart. If this is not done, then other members of the health care team may not be aware of what has happened. If there are any significant changes, be sure to speak directly to the patient's primary physician. Many institutions have a specific form that needs to be completed in the case of fall, but this does not take the place of good notes in the chart.

26 | Blood Pressure Changes

Markus J. Kraebber

When you are covering the wards, you often will be called because a patient's blood pressure is either high or low. This chapter focuses on blood pressure changes pertinent to psychiatric patients.

■ PHONE CALL

Questions

1. What are the patient's blood pressure and other vital signs? Are they outside of the usual range for that patient?
2. Does the patient have any other symptoms (e.g., dizziness, confusion, tremor, chest pain or discomfort, decreased level of consciousness, headache, rigidity)?
3. Does the patient have a history of hypertension? Is he or she taking an antihypertensive medication? Is there a history of hypotension? Have there been previous reactions to medications?
4. Does the patient have a history of alcohol or other substance use? When was the last use?
5. What medications is the patient taking? When was the last dose?

Orders

In general, you should see the patient before giving any medication orders. But you may want to ask the nurse to
1. Repeat the vitals while you are on your way.
2. Hold any medication that could further elevate or lower blood pressure until you have had a chance to assess the patient.

Inform RN

"Will arrive in . . . minutes."

If the patient is in any distress, you should see him or her quickly. If the patient is hypotensive and may be medically unstable, see him or her immediately.

■ ELEVATOR THOUGHTS

What are common causes of blood pressure changes in patients on psychiatric wards?
- Normal physiology
- Essential hypertension
- Medication side effects
- Substance use or withdrawal
- Drug withdrawal (e.g., abrupt withdrawal of some antihypertensives may cause rebound hypertension)
- Drug interactions (monoamine oxidase inhibitors are particularly dangerous)

■ MAJOR THREAT TO LIFE

Fortunately, a change in blood pressure is usually an early symptom. If the patient is also having cardiac symptoms, this is clearly a threat to life. If the patient has a headache and high blood pressure, potentially lethal cerebrovascular problems must be considered, including neurologic emergencies, such as an intracranial bleed.

Neuroleptic malignant syndrome (NMS) is another condition that may present a serious threat to life. Although the hallmark of NMS is rigidity, many symptoms may be more prominent in its early stages, such as hypotension, hypertension, and tachycardia. This is a dangerous side effect of antipsychotic medications that must be considered in any patient taking these medications for any length of time. If the condition seems life threatening, get additional help. The patient may require transfer to a medical ward where he or she can be watched more closely. The medical consultant should be involved from the beginning.

■ BEDSIDE

Quick Look Test

How does the patient look (comfortable, ill, in acute distress)?
This will give you a quick clue to the urgency of the situation. You must still perform a complete assessment.

Airway and Vital Signs

What is the blood pressure (BP)?
Retake the BP yourself in both arms using a sphygmomanometer (blood pressure gauge). Certain medical conditions produce unilateral differences in BP in their stable state. Im-

properly fitting blood pressure cuffs may produce false results. You may also want to check orthostatics at this time.

What are the heart rate and temperature?

These may serve as clues if you suspect substance-related problems.

How is the patient breathing?

Patients in cardiac distress may complain of difficulty breathing.

Chart Review

In addition, you should get the following information:
1. Has the patient been started on any medication recently?
2. What has the patient's blood pressure been like at other times today and at the same time on other days?
3. Was a urine toxicology screen or a blood alcohol test performed on admission?
4. Is the patient on a special diet?

Selective History

Although you may have found some of the answers to your questions in the chart or by talking to the nurse, you should also ask the patient directly. It is not uncommon for patients to forget to tell the doctor important information during the initial assessment.

Selective Physical Examination

1. **Vital signs:** If you have not already done so, take the vital signs now.
2. **General:** Is the patient in any distress or diaphoretic? What is the skin appearance?
3. **Lungs:** What is the respiratory rate? Are there crackles or wheezes?
4. **Cardiovascular:** Are there abnormal heart sounds? Is the rhythm regular? Is the heart rate abnormal?
5. **Neurologic:** What is the level of consciousness? Is there confusion or tremor? What is the tone?

■ MANAGEMENT

If the patient is in acute medical danger, alert the medical consultant immediately. Fortunately, most blood pressure changes will be relatively simple to handle. Sometimes when you take the BP yourself it will have normalized because it was just a physiologic elevation or decrease. If the blood pressure has not returned to normal, however, the following are some management suggestions.

Neuroleptic Malignant Syndrome

As mentioned, NMS may present very subtly. Signs of autonomic instability, including hypotension or hypertension, may be the initial clues to the diagnosis. If NMS is suspected:

- Stop the patient's antipsychotic medication.
- Draw the patient's blood for creatine kinase determination and a complete blood count.
- Contact the medical consultant, as transfer to a medical ward or intensive care unit may be indicated.
- Provide supportive care (e.g., cooling blankets, fluids).
- Retake the patient's temperature and other vital signs.

Hypertension

- One of the most common causes of hypertension, especially in newly admitted psychiatric patients, is alcohol withdrawal. Early signs include increased blood pressure, tachycardia, hyperthermia, and tremor. You should discuss alcohol intake with such a patient. Even if he or she denies or minimizes alcohol use, if you suspect withdrawal, you should treat to prevent progression.
- Keep in mind that several of the medications commonly used in psychiatric settings can cause blood pressure fluctuations (e.g., monoamine oxidase inhibitors [MAOIs] in patients who are noncompliant with the special tyramine diet). If you suspect that hypertension is a medication side effect, have that medication withheld until the assigned treatment team can make a decision on treatment options.
- If the patient has a history of high blood pressure and is taking an antihypertensive medication, ask the nurses when the last dose was given and when the next does is expected. Find out the usual range for this patient. You may want to give the next dose early. If the hypertension is mild and has been persistent, you should at least leave a note recommending that the dose be evaluated, a new medication tried, or a medical consultant called.
- If the patient has no history of high blood pressure and this is an isolated finding (no previous high readings and not now acute), have the patient's vital signs monitored regularly to watch for an impending problem. If there seems to be a pattern suggesting a new diagnosis of hypertension and the

patient's condition is not acute, you should leave a note recommending regular monitoring and that the patient be evaluated by an internist for medication. This option allows the treatment team to choose an appropriate antihypertensive. It is seldom necessary to start antihypertensive therapy as soon as possible. Unless there are signs of target organ damage, it is preferable to try nonpharmacologic modification for 4 to 6 weeks.

Hypotension

- The most common cause of hypotension in psychiatric patients (other than normal variations) is medication side effect.
- This frequently occurs upon the initiation of new medication or an increase in dose, but it can also occur in the patient who has been taking a medication for a while. Generally, patients will adapt to mild hypotension in time. If the patient is asymptomatic and tolerating the lowered blood pressure, you can simply monitor the patient's vital signs.
- Because many psychiatric medications may cause decreases in blood pressure, you will see this problem frequently. Use the information you gathered from the patient, chart, and nurses. If the patient is experiencing hypotension with mild symptoms (e.g., dizziness, light-headedness), withhold the next dose of the medications that you think might be causative. Write a note informing the treatment team of what you have done so that they can make appropriate subsequent decisions for the patient.
- Another cause of hypotension is dehydration. This may occur in depressed patients with decreased appetite, patients with eating disorders, or psychotic patients with delusions. If you suspect dehydration, check orthostatics and other vital signs to make sure that the patient is stable. If the patient appears stable, order laboratory tests. If you have any suspicion that the patient is not stable, draw samples for laboratory tests and send them yourself. Write orders to encourage fluid intake. If the patient is or becomes unstable, contact the medical consultant and arrange for transfer to a ward where the patient can receive the appropriate interventions.

■ REMEMBER

Always leave a note. Events that happened during the night often do not get reported during the morning rounds. If you had to see the patient, it is probably important enough for the treatment team to know about. The best course of action is to contact the treatment team yourself.

APPENDICES

APPENDIX A
Mini-Mental State Examination

Mini-Mental State Examination

I. ORIENTATION (*Ask the following questions; correct* = ⊠)   (Maximum score = 10)

What is today's date?	Date (e.g., May 21) 1
What is today's year?	Year 1
What is the month?	Month 1
What day is today?	Day (e.g., Monday) 1
Can you also tell me what season it is?	Season 1
Can you also tell me the name of this hospital/clinic?	Hospital/Clinic 1
What floor are we on?	Floor 1
What town/city are we in?	Town/City 1
What county are we in?	County 1
What state are we in?	State 1

II. IMMEDIATE RECALL (*correct* = ⊠)   (Maximum score = 3)

Ask the subject if you may test his or her memory. Say *"ball," "flag," "tree"* clearly and slowly, about one second for each. Then ask the subject to repeat them. Check the box at right for each correct response. The first repetition determines the score. If he or she does not repeat all three correctly, keep saying them up to six tries until he or she can repeat them.

Ball	 1
Flag	 1
Tree	 1
NUMBER OF TRIALS:	_____

III. ATTENTION AND CALCULATION (*Record each response; correct* = ⊠)   (Maximum final score = 5)

A. Counting Backward Test

Ask the subject to begin with 100 and count backward by 7. Record each response. Check one box at right for each correct response. Any response 7 less than the previous response is a correct response. The score is the number of correct subtractions. For example, 93, 87, 80, 73, 66 is a score of 4; 93, 86, 78, 70, 62 is 2; 92, 87, 78, 70, 65 is 0.

B. Spelling Backward Test

As the subject to spell the word "world" backward. Record each response. Use the instructions to determine which are correct responses, and check one box at right for each correct response.

C. Final Score

Compare the scores of the Counting Backward and Spelling Backward tests. Write the greater of the two scores in the box labeled **FINAL SCORE** at right, and use it in deriving the **TOTAL SCORE.**

RESPONSES	
93	1
86	1
79	1
72	1
65	1
D	1
L	1
R	1
O	1
W	1
FINAL SCORE	_____

IV. RECALL *(correct = ☒)*

Ask the subject to recall the three words you previously asked him or her to remember. Check the box at right for each correct response.

(Maximum score = 3)

Ball .... 1☐
Flag .... 1☐
Tree .... 1☐

V. LANGUAGE *(correct = ☒)*

(Maximum score = 9)

Naming
Show the subject a wrist watch and ask him or her what it is. Repeat for a pencil.

Watch .... 1☐
Pencil .... 1☐

Repetition
Ask the subject to repeat "No ifs, ands, or buts."

Repetition .... 1☐

Three-Stage Command
Establish the subject's dominant hand. Give the subject a sheet of blank paper and say, "Take the paper in your right/left hand, fold it in half, and put it on the floor."

Takes paper in hand .... 1☐
Folds paper in half .... 1☐
Puts paper on floor .... 1☐

Reading
Hold up a card that reads *"Close your eyes"* so the subject can see it clearly. Ask him or her to read it and do what it says. Check the box at right only if he or she actually closes his or her eyes.

Closes eyes ...... 1☐

Writing
Give the subject a sheet of blank paper and ask him or her to write a sentence. It is to be written spontaneously. If the sentence contains a subject and a verb, and is sensible, check the box at right. Correct grammar and punctuation are not necessary.

Writes sentence ...... 1☐

Copying
Show the subject the drawing of intersecting pentagons. Ask him or her to draw the pentagons (about one inch each side) on paper provided. If 10 angles are present and 2 intersect, check the box at right. Ignore tremor and rotation.

Copies pentagons .... 1☐

DERIVING THE TOTAL SCORE

Add the number of correct responses. The maximum score is 30.

TOTAL SCORE ☐

Reprinted from Folstein MF, Folstein SE, McHugh PR: Mini-mental state: A practical method for grading the cognitive state of patients for the clinician. Journal of Psychiatric Research 12:189–198, 1975. © 1975, 1998 MiniMental LLC.

Close your eyes

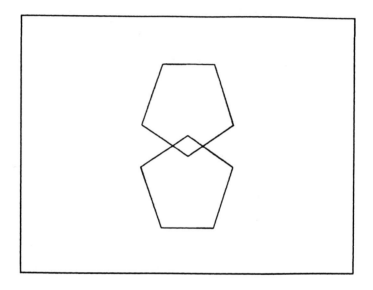

APPENDIX B
Mental Status Examination

NOAH L. ROSEN
SIDDHARTHA NADKARNI

During the evaluation of a patient, the history is obtained in order to answer the question: What has happened that has brought the patient here? It does not directly answer the question: Who is the patient? That is the purpose of the mental status examination (MSE). The MSE is an organized compilation of the psychiatrist's subjective and objective observations of the patient. Remember that the MSE provides a "snapshot" of the psychologic life of the patient and will therefore supply other people with the description of how the patient was **at the time of evaluation.** Specific questions must be asked, and the gestalt of the interview should be quantified. The examination is divided into 16 major categories, all of which should be included. The various subcategories need be reported only if there are significant positives or negatives.

1. General appearance
    Overall appearance
    Grooming
    Posture
    Facial expression
    Emotional appearance (e.g., anxious, tense, panicky, sad, unhappy, angry)
2. Speech
    Rate (e.g., slow, fast, pressured, interruptible)
    Quality (e.g., faint, hoarse)
    Spontaneity
    Stammering or stuttering
    Slurring
    Articulation (may test *k*, *t*, and *m* sounds for localizing weak musculature)
    Pitch
    Prosody: emotional intonation (a nondominant hemisphere–mediated ability)
    Aphasia: impaired communication by speech, writing, or signs due to dysfunction of the brain centers in dominant hemisphere (see Appendix D for more details)
    Paraphasia: word interposition and substitution causing unintelligible speech
    Neologism: use of a word in a novel or incorrect manner
    Clang associations: use of words similar in sound but not in meaning
    Echolalia: involuntary repetition of a phrase spoken by another person
    Muteness: lack of speech

3. Attitude: the way of thinking, feeling, or acting toward a situation (e.g., irritable, aggressive, seductive, guarded, defensive, indifferent, cooperative, sarcastic)
4. Motor behavior
   Level of activity (e.g., psychomotor agitation or retardation)
   Tics or tremors
   Automatisms: involuntarily performed movements
   Mannerisms
   Grimacing
   Gestures
   Stereotypy: constant repetition of a meaningless gesture
   Apraxia: inability to voluntarily perform a specific purposeful movement or utilize a known object
   Gait
   Akathisia: inability to remain seated due to motor restlessness
   Dyskinesia: insuppressible, stereotyped, awake-state involuntary movements
5. Mood: the patient's subjective experience of his or her emotional state (e.g., gloomy, sad/depressed, angry, tense, euphoric, happy)
6. Affect: the evaluator's observations of the patient's emotional state
   Quality (e.g., labile, blunted, constricted, flat, euphoric)
   Mood congruity and appropriateness
   Range and intensity
7. Thought process
   Quality (e.g., logical, sequential, goal-directed, circumstantial, tangential, flight of ideas, looseness of association)
   Relevance
   Clang associations
   Perseveration
8. Thought content
   Suicidal or homicidal ideation: be specific about degree of intent, previous attempts, and any planning
   Delusions: always note specific details and how well formed they appear (e.g., persecution, grandiosity, infidelity, somatic, sensory)
   Thought broadcasting or insertion
   Ideas of reference: false belief that an occurrence carries special meaning relating to oneself
   Phobia: objectively unfounded morbid dread or fear
   Preoccupation
   Obsession: an anxiety condition in which one idea constantly fills the mind
   Compulsion: uncontrollable impulse to perform an act, often repetitively
   Thought blocking
   Depersonalization: feeling of losing identity or disconnection from reality
   Magical thinking
9. Perceptual disorders
   Hallucinations: subjective experiences without basis in reality (e.g., olfactory, auditory, tactile, gustatory, visual)
   Illusions: misperceptions of real experiences

Hypnopompic or hypnagogic experiences: hallucinations that occur in the transitional state between sleeping and waking

Feelings of unreality

Déjà vu: mental impression that a new experience has happened before

Jamais vu: false feeling of unfamiliarity with a familiar experience

Time loss and amnesia

10. Sensorium

Level of arousal (e.g., alert, lethargic, obtunded, stuporous, comatose)

Orientation to person, place, time, and situation

Cognition and abstraction

11. Mini-mental status examination

This should be used as a basic indicator for deficits of orientation, memory, attention, calculation, and language. The full examination appears in Appendix A. Any impairment should be further evaluated and described in the other categories of the mental status examination.

12. Memory

Remote: may test by asking basic knowledge questions (e.g., Who was the first President?)

Recent: may test by asking questions about current events or major news stories

Immediate: may test with 3-word immediate recall and 5-minute retest

13. Concentration and calculations

Ability to pay attention: may test with serial 7 subtractions or naming the days of the week or the months of the year backwards

Distractibility

14. Information and intelligence

Use of vocabulary

Level of education

Fund of knowledge

15. Judgment: the ability to form sound opinions and demonstrate good sense

Ability to understand facts

Capability of manipulating data

Facility for drawing and relating conclusions

16. Insight: understanding, especially of one's own condition (e.g., poor, limited, fair, good)

APPENDIX C

Medical Conditions Manifesting as Psychiatric Disorders

STEVEN WOZNIAK

The following table lists medical disorders that are commonly associated with psychiatric symptoms, with an emphasis on those disorders that are most often considered in the psychiatric differential diagnosis.

Disorder	Common Medical Complaints	Psychiatric Presentation	Diagnostic Tests	Comments
Acute intermittent porphyria	Abdominal pain, nausea, vomiting, peripheral neuropathy, constipation, tachycardia, hypertension, seizures	Anxiety, insomnia, depression, psychosis, delirium	Urine porphyrins, Watson-Schwartz or Hoesch test	Autosomal dominant; attacks may be induced by medications, diet
Adrenal cortical insufficiency (e.g., Addison's disease)	Hyperpigmentation, orthostatic hypotension, anorexia, dizziness, weakness	Depression	Serum and urine cortisol, serum aldosterone and renin, serum and urine sodium, serum potassium, abdominal CT	Multiple causes
AIDS	Fever, weight loss, lymphadenopathy, neurologic changes	Anxiety, depression, psychosis, dementia	HIV serology and Western blot; consider imaging and CSF studies	
Anemia	Dyspnea on exertion, dizziness, lightheadedness, palpitations, syncope	Mood changes, poor concentration, worsening of dementia	CBC, blood smear, reticulocyte count, iron and vitamin B_{12}, folate	
Any cancer	Various	Depression, anxiety	Tests depend on etiology	May be reactive depression

Table continued on following page

Disorder	Common Medical Complaints	Psychiatric Presentation	Diagnostic Tests	Comments
Arsenic poisoning	Abdominal pain, GI symptoms, headache, weakness; chronic exposure: hyperpigmentation, hepatic disease, alopecia	Delirium, psychosis	Urine heavy metal screen	Occupational exposure common
Chronic hypoxia	Possibly evidence of congestive heart failure	Confusion, fatigue	Arterial blood gas, pulmonary function tests, chest x-ray	Multiple causes
Chronic renal failure	Peripheral neuropathy, signs of multisystem disease	Fatigue, mood changes, irritability	Serum electrolytes, CBC, urinalysis, renal imaging	Diabetes mellitus and hypertension most common causes
Cryptococcal meningitis	Headache, nausea, vomiting, seizures, ataxia, ocular changes	Personality change, confusion, lethargy, dementia	Head MRI or CT, CSF and serum cryptococcal antigen	Occurs in 5–10% of HIV-infected patients; insidious onset
Giant cell arteritis (temporal arteritis)	Headache, joint and muscle pain, fever, vision loss, jaw claudication, polymyalgia rheumatica	Depression, confusion, psychosis	Temporal artery biopsy, ESR	Rapid diagnosis and treatment may prevent blindness
Hepatic encephalopathy	Ataxia, asterixis, seizures, fetor hepaticus	Mood and sleep changes, agitation, confusion	Liver function tests, ammonia level	Avoid alcohol and hepatotoxic medications

Disorder	Physical Findings	Psychiatric Manifestations	Diagnostic Tests	Comments
Hepatolenticular degeneration [Wilson's disease]	Abdominal pain, hepatitis, Kayser-Fleischer rings, hemolytic anemia	Mood and personality changes, psychosis, dementia	Serum and urinary copper; ceruloplasmin, slit-lamp examination	Autosomal recessive
Hyperadrenalism [Cushing's syndrome]	Central obesity, moon facies, striae, weakness, acne, hypertension, diabetes, osteoporosis	Depression, mood lability, psychosis	Serum and urine cortisol, dexamethasone suppression test, imaging studies	Most common cause is iatrogenic
Hypercalcemia	Weakness, fatigue, constipation, anorexia, nausea, dyspepsia, polyuria, renal stones, soft-tissue calcification, QT interval shortening	Depression, confusion	Serum calcium and parathyroid hormone	Multiple causes
Hypernatremia	Respiratory paralysis, seizures	Somnolence, confusion, coma	Serum and urine sodium and osmolality	
Hyperparathyroidism	Hypercalcemia, weight loss, constipation, dyspepsia, renal stones, proximal muscle weakness, bone pain	Depression, anxiety, confusion, irritability, psychosis	Serum calcium, phosphorus, and parathyroid hormone; bone radiographs	
Hyperthyroidism [thyrotoxicosis]	Tremor, weight loss, palpitations, warm moist skin, hair loss, weakness, malaise	Anxiety, depression, irritability, insomnia, psychosis	Thyroid hormones, thyroid stimulation test, imaging studies	Rapid onset, resembles anxiety; slow onset, depression

Table continued on following page

Disorder	Common Medical Complaints	Psychiatric Presentation	Diagnostic Tests	Comments
Hypoparathyroidism	Hypocalcemia, dry skin, diarrhea, congestive heart failure, extrapyramidal symptoms, tetany, numbness, tingling	Irritability, paranoia, depression, psychosis	Serum calcium, phosphorus, and parathyroid hormone	Iatrogenic (postsurgical) most common
Hypothyroidism (myxedema)	Dry skin, coarse hair, cold intolerance, weight gain, anorexia	Fatigue, depression, anxiety, psychosis, personality change	Thyroid hormones, thyroid stimulation test, imaging studies	Slow onset resembles depression or sleep apnea
Intracranial tumor	Headache, vomiting, focal neurologic findings, papilledema	Personality and mood changes, psychosis, dementia	LP opening pressure, head CT or MRI	
Ischemic heart disease	Chest pain, heart failure, myocardial infarction	Anxiety, panic, depression	Chest x-ray, electrocardiogram, stress test, coronary arteriography	Must differentiate from anxiety without cardiac disease
Lead poisoning	Abdominal pain, GI symptoms, headache, seizures, focal neurologic signs	Irritability, delirium, dementia	Serum and urine lead, blood smear for basophilic stippling, bone lead levels	Children and persons with paint and industrial exposures most commonly affected
Mercury poisoning	Tremor, GI distress, dermatitis, sensorimotor impairments	Fatigue, anxiety, irritability, depression	Serum and urine mercury levels	

Mitral valve prolapse	Usually asymptomatic, arrhythmias, chest pain	Anxiety, panic	Electrocardiogram	More common in women
Multiple sclerosis	Waxing and waning focal neurologic deficits, paresthesias, optic neuritis	Mood changes, chronic fatigue, memory impairment	White matter lesions on MRI, CSF assay for gamma globulins and oligoclonal bands	May be mistaken for somatization
Neurosyphilis	Headache, vertigo, hyperreflexia, Argyll Robertson pupils, stroke, ataxia, bladder disturbances	Insomnia, mood and personality changes, psychosis, dementia	CSF serology	
Normal-pressure hydrocephalus	Abnormal gait, urinary incontinence, dementia	Dementia, psychomotor retardation, apathy	Head CT or MRI	A treatable cause of dementia
Pancreatic carcinoma	Abdominal pain, weight loss, anorexia, nausea, vomiting	Depression, lethargy	Abdominal imaging, ERCP	Insidious onset
Pheochromo-cytoma	Hypertension, paroxysmal headache, sweating, palpitations, tachycardia	Anxiety, panic	24-hour urine assay for catecholamines, metanephrines, and vanillylmandelic acid	May have family history of disorder
Seizure disorder (epilepsy)	Episodic staring, tonic-clonic jerking, sensory aura, automatisms	Memory problems, mood and personality changes, illusions and hallucinations	Electroencephalogram	

Table continued on following page

Disorder	Common Medical Complaints	Psychiatric Presentation	Diagnostic Tests	Comments
Subdural hematoma	Headache, focal weakness	Irritability, confusion, hypersomnolence, dementia	Head CT or MRI	Precipitating trauma may be minor or not remembered
Systemic lupus erythematosus	Arthritis, malar rash, lymphadenopathy, oral ulcers, weight loss, photosensitivity	Depression, fatigue, psychosis, mania	ESR, ANA, serum complement levels	Female predominance 10 to 1; corticosteroid treatment may complicate psychiatric features
Thiamine deficiency	Neuropathy, ophthalmoplegia, Wernicke-Korsakoff syndrome	Amnesia, confabulation, confusion	Thiamine level	Common in alcoholic patients
Tuberculous meningitis	Fever, weight loss, headache, SIADH, meningeal signs	Lethargy, confusion, obtundation	CSF assay for cells, protein, glucose, acid-fast bacteria; CSF cultures	
Vitamin B_{12} deficiency	Ataxia, peripheral neuropathy, GI symptoms	Mood changes, anxiety, psychosis, dementia, fatigue	Serum B_{12} and folate, red cell indices, Schilling's test	Pernicious anemia a common cause

Data from Goldman L, Bennett JC (eds): Cecil Textbook of Medicine, 21st Edition. Philadelphia, WB Saunders, 2000; Fauci AS, Braunwald EB, Isselbacher KJ, et al (eds). Harrison's Principles of Internal Medicine, 14th Edition. New York, McGraw-Hill, 1998; Wyszynski AA, Wyszynski B: A Case Approach to Medical-Psychiatric Practice. Washington, DC, American Psychiatric Press, 1996; Jenkins SC, Hansen MR: A Pocket Reference for Psychiatrists, 2nd Edition. Washington, DC, American Psychiatric Press, 1995, pp 76–88.

APPENDIX D
The Neurologic Examination

Siddhartha Nadkarni
Noah L. Rosen

The neurologic examination provides a means to obtain singular information, namely, whether a patient's nervous system is working or not
and, if not, where the problem may lie. A directed neurologic examination
is indispensible for certain on-call situations and even as a screen for
patients to be admitted to an inpatient service. It can be done swiftly and
does not always need to cover all the details below. Rather, it may be
guided by the patient's history. It is an invaluable tool to help stratify
priorities in the middle of the night.

The neurologic examination consists of the following:

Mental status
Cranial nerves
Motor
Sensory
Coordination
Gait
Reflexes

The italicized terms in parentheses in this appendix indicate the most
likely localizations for the deficits elicited by the tested function.

MENTAL STATUS

The part of the neurologic examination concerned with mental status
is similar to the formal mental status examination described in Appendix
B but with a concentration on six **realms**.

Level of Consciousness

You should describe the patient's best response to verbal, tactile, or
painful/noxious stimuli. Note if the patient is awake/alert,
hypersomnolent/drowsy/lethargic, stuporous (responds to painful stimuli), or comatose (no response to painful stimuli). You may use the
Glasgow Coma Scale measuring three parameters and assessing points
in each:

Eye opening (spontaneous, 4; to voice, 3; to pain, 2; none, 1)
Best motor response (obeys commands, 6; localizes to pain, 5; with-
draws to pain, 4; flexor posturing, 3; extensor posturing, 2; none, 1)
Best verbal response (conversant and oriented, 5; conversant and disori-

ented, 4; uses inappropriate words, 3; makes incomprehensible sounds, 2; none, 1)

Make sure to note what the patient missed and to take into account underlying psychopathology. *(brain stem, bilateral cerebral)*

Orientation

Person: governor, mayor, president, spouse, **not self**
Place: type (hospital), name, city, floor, county
Time: day, date with year, time of day, season
Situation (related to insight)
General current events
(frontal, temporal lobes)

Memory

Name three objects and have the patient repeat them out loud one or two times. After 5 minutes, ask the patient to repeat the three objects; if the patient is unsuccessful, you may give multiple choice or other cues. Normally a person should not need any cues. *(mesial temporal, hippocampi)*

Language

Naming: Ask the patient to name both high frequency (watch, table, pen, door) and low frequency (watchband, clasp, lapel, cuff) words.
Fluency: Is the patient speaking swiftly with normal volume and flow of words, or is there a paucity of words and frustration in getting them out?
Comprehension: Can the patient follow commands and understand what is said?
Repetition: Can the patient repeat short phrases or sentences ("no ifs, ands, or buts" and "today is a sunny day" or "the spy fled to Greece")?
Other areas of language: Does the patient use paraphasic errors, clang associations, or inappropriate syntax, diction, prosody, rate of speech, volume of speech?

Aphasia	Fluency	Comprehension	Naming	Repetition
Broca's (expressive), motor	−	+	−	−
Wernicke's (receptive), motor	+	−	−	−
Transcortical, motor	−	+	−	+
Transcortical, sensory	+	−	−	+
Global	−	−	−	−
Conduction	+	+	+	−
Anomic	+	+	−	+

− = Abnormal; + = normal.
(frontal, temporal, deep white matter)

Attention/Concentration

Test by having the patient cite numbers serially by sevens, name the months backward (not related to education as much), spell w-o-r-l-d backward, or cite a string of numbers backward or forward (6 to 7 forward and 4 to 5 backward is normal). *(frontal)*

Higher Cognitive Functions

Thought content/process, abstraction, insight, judgment, mood, and affect are all discussed earlier.

Praxis: the ability to execute learned/commanded behavior—such as "brush teeth" or "comb hair" *(dominant parietal)*

Visuospatial orientation: drawing Rey diagram or pentagons/clock, cardinal directions *(nondominant parietal)*

Left-right confusion/crossing midline: "touch left ear with right thumb" *(dominant parietotemporal)*

CRANIAL NERVES

I Olfactory: Test smell with non-noxious agents, especially for head trauma. *(frontal)*

II Optic: Test for visual acuity *(optic nerve, occipital cortex, lens, retina)* and visual fields (very important; *retina, optic nerve, optic chiasm, optic tracts, lateral geniculate bodies, optic radiations, occipital lobes)* in each eye separately, both nasal and temporal and superior and inferior. Also test for direct pupillary response.

III Oculomotor: This nerve is responsible for all extraocular movements except down-and-out and abduction. Look for ptosis (drooping of an eyelid) and miosis (small, poorly reactive pupil). (Horner's syndrome is ptosis, miosis, and anhidrosis from disruption of sympathetic pathways centrally or peripherally. *(midbrain or third cranial nerve)*

IV Trochlear: This nerve moves the eyes down and out. *(midbrain)*

V Trigeminal: The trigeminal nerve is sensory in three divisions (V1, V2, V3) to the face. Use the pin/light touch test, evaluate motor function (muscles of mastication, masseters/pterygoid) and reflexes (afferent of corneal and responsible for jaw jerk). *(pons)*

VI Abducens: Test the patient's abduction of the eyes. *(false localizer, pontomedullary junction)*

VII Facial: This nerve innervates the muscles of facial expression. Ask the patient to smile and raise eyebrows. If the forehead is involved, the lesion is peripheral; if only the lower face is involved, the lesion is central. *(cerebellopontine angle, VIIth nerve)*

VIII Vestibulocochlear: This nerve is responsible for hearing and vestibulo-ocular reflexes. Whisper multisyllabic words in each ear or rub the fingers by each ear with the patient's eyes closed. *(cerebellopontine angle, VIIIth nerve)*

IX Glossopharyngeal: This nerve raises the palate and is responsible for the gag reflex. Have the patient open the mouth wide and say "aah." The uvula points to the side of the lesion. *(medulla)*

   X Vagus: This nerve is responsible and testable for the same functions as cranial nerve IX, and also for autonomic functions. *(medulla)*

  XI Spinal accessory: Have the patient shrug the shoulder and turn the head, and look for weakness. *(medulla)*

 XII Hypoglossal: This nerve is responsible for motor function of the tongue. Have the patient stick the tongue out and move it from side to side. The tongue tends to point to the side of the lesion and is slower or weaker in movements on the ipsilateral side of the lesion. *(medulla)*

MOTOR

Graded system: 5/5, normal full strength; 4/5, against resistance but not fully (may be 4+ or 4−); 3/5, against gravity but not resistance; 2/5, not against gravity but can move in plane perpendicular to vector of gravity; 1/5, flicker of contraction but no movement; 0/5, no contraction. Always compare one side with the other for each muscle at the time it is tested. Test for tone/tremor.

Confrontational testing: deltoids, biceps, triceps, wrist flexors/extensors, intrinsic hand muscles, iliopsoas (hip flexion), gluteus maximus (hip extension), quadriceps, hamstrings, thigh abductors/adductors, tibialis anterior (dorsiflexion/inversion of foot), gastrocnemius/soleus (plantarflexion of foot/toes), peronei (eversion of foot)

Subtle testing for weakness: pronator drift of outstretched arms with palms up, fine finger movements, heel and toe walking, hopping on one foot *(peripheral nerve, plexus, nerve root, spinal cord, brain stem, internal capsule, corona, frontal)*

SENSORY

There are four modalities: pain/temperature (pinprick), light touch, position/vibration, and cortical (double simultaneous extinction [tactile/visual/auditory], stereognosis, graphesthesia). *(peripheral nerve, plexus, nerve root, spinal cord, brain stem, thalamus, parietal)*

COORDINATION

Test finger-nose-finger, rapid alternating movements, and heel-knee-shin for dysmetria. Test Romberg's sign, and look for nystagmus. *(spinocerebellar tracts in spinal cord, cerebellum, thalamus, basal ganglia)*

GAIT

Test stance and walk, noting foot excursion off the ground, length and sureness of stride, ataxia, initiation, turning, and tandem (tight-rope walking). *(May be multifactorial with contributors from nearly any of the systems above)*

REFLEXES

Graded system: 0, no reflex; 1+, hyporeflexia; 2+, normal; 3+, hyper-reflexia possibly with unsustained clonus; 4+, marked hyperreflexia possibly with sustained clonus. Always compare both sides before moving to the next reflex.

Deep tendon reflexes: biceps, triceps, brachioradialis, patellar, Achilles

Superficial reflexes: abdominal (stroke lightly on the abdomen), cremasteric, plantar (Babinski: big toe goes up and rest of toes fan out)

Other: finger flexors (hyperreflexia if fingers have exaggerated flexion when tapped lightly on the palmar surface), Hoffman's (hyperreflexia if thumb and forefinger flex when flicking the nail of the middle finger), jaw jerk (if exaggerated, will place lesion at the level of cranial nerve V in the brain stem or above)

Frontal release signs: primitive reflexes are often seen if the frontal lobe is involved; glabellar (with tapping on forehead, patient cannot stop blinking even if asked); palmomental (stroking palm produces flexion of ipsilateral mentalis muscle); forced grasp (placing fingers between thumb and first finger, patient will grasp); root (patient will move lips to stimulus at corner of mouth); snout (tapping slightly on lips produces puckering)

NOTES

For upper motor neuron signs (hyperreflexia, Babinski, spastic weakness), place the lesion above the conus medullaris of the spinal cord and in the central nervous system. For lower motor neuron signs (hyporeflexia, fasciculations, flaccid weakness), place the lesion distal to the conus or cord in the case of root or plexus lesions.

Depending on the patient's history and situation, brief screens can be used to elicit findings such as drift and double simultaneous extinction.

APPENDIX E
Normal Laboratory Values

ERWIN C. TING

Complete blood count	
Erythrocytes	$4.2–5.6 \times 10^6/\mu L$
Hemoglobin	Male: 13.6–17.5 g/dL
	Female: 120–155 g/dL
Hematocrit	Male: 0.39–0.49
	Female: 0.35–0.45
Mean corpuscular hemoglobin	26–34 pg
Mean corpuscular hemoglobin	31–36 g/dL
concentration	
Mean corpuscular volume	80–100 fL
Platelets	$150–450 \times 10^3/\mu L$
Reticulocytes	$33–137 \times 10^3/\mu L$
White blood cells	$4.8–10.8 \times 10^9/L$
Electrolytes (serum)	
Bicarbonate	22–28 mEq/L
Blood urea nitrogen (BUN)	8–20 mEq/L
Calcium	8.5–10.5 mg/dL
Chloride	98–107 mEq/L
Creatinine	0.6–1.2 mEq/L
Glucose	60–115 mg/dL
Magnesium	1.8–3.0 mg/dL
Phosphorus	2.5–4.5 mg/dL
Potassium	3.5–5.0 mEq/L
Sodium	135–145 mEq/L
Liver function tests	
Alanine aminotransferase (ALT)	0–35 U/L
Albumin	3.4–4.7 g/dL
Alkaline phosphatase	41–133 U/L
Aspartate transaminase (AST)	0–35 U/L
Bilirubin	
Direct	0.1–0.4 mg/dL
Indirect	0.1–0.7 mg/dL
Total	0.1–1.2 mg/dL
Lactate dehydrogenase	88–230 U/L
Total protein	6.0–8.0 g/dL
Thyroid function tests	
Thyroid-stimulating hormone	$0.4–6 \mu U/mL$
Thyroxine, total (T_4)	$5–11 \mu g/dL$
Triiodothyronine, total (T_3)	95–190 ng/dL
Thyroxine, free (fT_4)	9–24 pmol/L
Amylase	20–110 U/L

Ammonia	18–60 μg/dL
Acetoacetate	Negative
Ceruloplasmin	20–35 mg/dL
Cholesterol	<200 mg/dL
Cortisol	8:00 AM: 5–20 μg/dL
Ethanol	<80 mg/dL
Fibrin D-dimer	Negative
Fibrinogen	175–433 mg/dL
Lactic acid (lactate)	0.5–2.0 mEq/L
Lipase	0–160 U/L
Partial thromboplastin time, activated (PTT)	25–30 sec
Prothrombin time (PT)	11–15 sec
International Normalized Ratio (INR)	2–3.5
Triglyceride	<165 mg/dL
Vitamin B_{12}	140–820 pg/mL

Note: Normal values may vary from institution to institution. Check with your own laboratory to verify its reference ranges.

APPENDIX F
Urine Toxicology

JONATHAN BELLMAN

Drug	Screening Cut-off Concentration (ng/mL)	Urine Detection Time*
Alcohol	300,000	7–12 hours
Amphetamine	1000	2–4 days
Barbiturates		
Short-acting	200	2–4 days
Long-acting	200	Up to 30 days
Benzodiazepines	200	Up to 30 days
Cocaine	300	1–3 days
Codeine	300	1–3 days
Heroin	300	1–3 days
Marijuana	50 (varies by laboratory)	Casual use, 1–3 days Chronic use, up to 30 days
Methadone	300	2–4 days
Methamphetamine	1000	2–4 days
Phencyclidine	25	Casual use, 2–7 days Chronic use, up to 30 days

*May vary widely depending on amount ingested, compound, physical state of subject, and other factors.

Although ingestion of some foods and medications may result in positive preliminary tests, most medical centers utilize alternative methods to confirm positive screening results. Gas chromatography–mass spectrometry (GC-MS) is the most reliable, most definitive procedure for drug identification.

The following should be kept in mind when certain test results are interpreted:

Ibuprofen was found to interfere with the Syva EMIT test and to cause apparent false-positive results for the marijuana metabolite. Syva has corrected the problem by altering the formulation of the EMIT kit.

Phenylpropanolamine (PPA) and ephedrine, found in over-the-counter (OTC) diet pills and cold remedies, are similar in chemical structure to amphetamines and can produce a false-positive result for amphetamines in immunoassay screens.

Ibuprofen, PPA, and ephedrine preparations will not lead to a false-positive error if an appropriate GC-MS confirmation assay is carried out because the GC-MS technique can specifically identify the illicit drug.

Poppy seeds cause true-positive results for opioids because there can be sufficient morphine in the seeds to be detected in the urine. The amount is seldom, however, above the screening cut-off concentration.

APPENDIX G
Medication Levels

JONATHAN BELLMAN

Drug	Dose Range	Plasma Range
Antidepressants		
Amitriptyline	50–300 mg/day	80–250 ng/mL
Nortriptyline	30–125 mg/day	50–150 ng/mL
Imipramine	50–300 mg/day	150–250 ng/mL
Desipramine	50–300 mg/day	125–300 ng/mL
Mood stabilizers		
Lithium	1200–1800 mg/day	0.8–1.3 mEq/L
Carbamazepine	600–1600 mg/day	4–12 μg/mL
Valproic acid	750–2500 mg/day	50–100 ng/mL

APPENDIX H

Clonidine Detoxification Protocol for Opioid Dependence

M. BREALYN SELLERS
SCOTT BIENENFELD

Day 1	0.1–0.2 mg orally in three divided doses or every 4 hours up to 1.0 mg
Days 2–4	0.1–0.2 mg orally in three divided doses or every 4 hours up to 1.0 mg
Day 5 to completion	Reduce 0.2 mg per day in three divided doses; reduce the nighttime dose last or reduce by one-half each day, not to exceed 0.4 mg per day

Adapted from Kleber HD: Detoxification from narcotics. In Lowinson JH, Ruiz P (eds): Substance Abuse: Clinical Issues and Perspectives. Baltimore, Williams & Wilkins, 1981, pp 317–339.

APPENDIX I

Detoxification Protocol for Alcohol Dependence

SCOTT BIENENFELD
M. BREALYN SELLERS

Administer chlordiazepoxide in tapered dosages as follows:
  Chlordiazepoxide 50 mg PO every 6 hours for 4 doses
  Chlordiazepoxide 25 mg PO every 6 hours for 4 doses
  Chlordiazepoxide 10 mg PO every 6 hours for 4 doses
  Chlordiazepoxide 25 mg or 50 mg PO every 6 hours PRN for
    breakthrough withdrawal
If the patient has hepatic impairment or PO access is not available,
    use lorazepam in tapered dosages as follows:
  Lorazepam 2 mg PO/IM every 4–6 hours for 4 doses
  Lorazepam 1 mg PO/IM every 4–6 hours for 4 doses
  Lorazepam 0.5 mg PO/IM every 4–6 hours for 4 doses
  Lorazepam 2 mg PO every 4 hours PRN for breakthrough
    withdrawal
Other medications may be given as follows:
  Thiamine 100 mg PO every day
  Folate 1 mg PO every day
  Vitamin B complex 1 tablet PO every day
  Ibuprofen 400 mg PO every 6 hours as needed for pain
  Diphenhydramine 50 mg or trazodone (Desyrel) 50 mg PO QHS
    PRN for insomnia

APPENDIX J
Admission Orders

Van Yu

Admit to
  Psychiatry, detoxification
  Specify unit
  Legal status (e.g., voluntary, involuntary, informal)
Diagnosis
  Axis I, II, III, IV, and V
Condition
  Stable, guarded
Vital signs
  Unit routine, every 4 hours
Allergy
Activity
  One-to-one observation, restraints, room restriction, as tolerated
Diet
  Regular, low salt, low cholesterol, 1800 calorie ADA, 3000 calorie
Laboratory tests
  Electrolyte panel, serum glucose, BUN, creatinine, liver function
    tests, TSH, CBC with differential, RPR (or VDRL), urinalysis, urine
    toxicology, ECG
  Consider: beta-HCG, T_4, vitamin B_{12}, folate, ESR, ANA, rheumatoid
    factor, medication levels (e.g., lithium level), serum alcohol,
    serum toxicology, chest x-ray, brain imaging (e.g., noncontrast
    head CT), EEG
Medications
  PRN medications (e.g., haloperidol 5 mg IM/PO every 2–8 hours
    and/or lorazepam 2 mg IM/PO every 2–8 hours)
  Standing medications

APPENDIX K

Common Adverse Effects of Psychotropic Medications

Sharon Falco
Christine Desmond

ANTIDEPRESSANT MEDICATIONS

Chemical Class and Drug	Adverse Effects							
	Neurologic	Dermatologic	Cardiovascular	Digestive	Endocrine	Hematologic	Ocular	Other
1. Selective serotonin reuptake inhibitors (SSRIs)								
Fluoxetine (Prozac)	Headache,‡ anxiety,‡ insomnia, drowsiness, fatigue, dizziness, tremor, sedation, seizures [12/6000 patients], extrapyramidal symptoms, akathisia	Pruritus, rash, diaphoresis	Slight sinus bradycardia, orthostatic hypotension 1%	Nausea/vomiting,† diarrhea, anorexia, dry mouth, dyspepsia, weight loss	Hypoglycemia,* hyperglycemia, hypothyroidism 1%, SIADH leading to hyponatremia	Anemia 1%	Visual impairment, blurred vision	Upper respiratory tract infection 8%, pharyngitis, nasal congestion, sinusitis, cough, dyspnea, increased urinary frequency 2%, sexual dysfunction‡ [20–50%], decreased libido,‡ delayed ejaculation, impotence, anorgasmia, spontaneous or delayed orgasm

Sertraline (Zoloft)	Insomnia,† drowsiness, dizziness,† tremor,† somnolence, fatigue, agitation, headache	Rash 2%, diaphoresis 8%	Palpitations 4%	Nausea/vomiting,† diarrhea,† dyspepsia,† dry mouth,† constipation, anorexia, abdominal cramps, dysgeusia (taste perversion) 1%, asymptomatic elevated hepatic enzymes 1%	Transient SIADH leading to hyponatremia	Blurred vision 4%	Sexual dysfunction,‡ ejaculatory delay 16%, anorgasmia 2%, increased urinary output
Paroxetine (Paxil)	Asthenia,‡ somnolence,‡ headache, dizziness,† insomnia,† tremor, paresthesias, hypotension	Diaphoresis,† rash, urticaria, erythema nodosum 1.7%, pruritus, alopecia, xerosis, angioedema (rare)	Palpitations 2.9%, orthostatic hypotension 1%, vasodilation 2.6%	Nausea/vomiting,‡ xerostomia,† constipation,† diarrhea,† anorexia, dyspepsia, flatulence, appetite stimulation, taste perversion, dry mouth	Hyponatremia	Visual impairment 3.6%	Pharyngitis, lump in throat, tightness in throat, increased urinary frequency, dysuria, sexual dysfunction,† anorgasmia, impotence, delayed ejaculation,† decreased libido
Fluvoxamine (Luvox)	Sedation,‡ headache, anxiety, nervousness, insomnia, drowsiness, fatigue, dizziness, tremor, asthenia, akathisia, dystonia	Diaphoresis 2%, toxic epidermal necrolysis (rare)	Sinus tachycardia (rare), palpitations (rare)	Nausea/vomiting,‡ dry mouth,† diarrhea, constipation,‡ dyspepsia, abdominal pain, anorexia	SIADH		Impotence, anorgasmia, increased urinary frequency 3%

Table continued on following page

ANTIDEPRESSANT MEDICATIONS *Continued*

Chemical Class and Drug	Adverse Effects							
	Neurologic	Dermatologic	Cardiovascular	Digestive	Endocrine	Hematologic	Ocular	Other
Citalopram (Celexa)	Paresthesia, migraine, sedation	Rash	Tachycardia, postural hypotension	Hypersalivation, flatulence, weight gain/loss, nausea				Decreased libido, impotence, anorgasmia, delayed ejaculation, coughing
2. Serotonin-norepinephrine reuptake inhibitors								
Venlafaxine (Effexor)	Sedation, ‡ drowsiness, † dizziness, † insomnia 18%, asthenia 12%, nervousness 13%, anxiety 6%, tremor 5%	Diaphoresis 12%	Dose-related hypertension in >5% of patients taking above 200 mg/day, changes in heart rate, sinus tachycardia in overdose	Nausea/vomiting, ‡ dry mouth 22%, constipation 15%, anorexia 11%, about 5% weight loss in 6% of patients			Blurred vision 6%	Decreased libido 2%, ejaculation dysfunction 12%, impotence 6%, orgasm disturbance, menstrual disorders

3. Tricyclics and tetracyclics Imipramine [Tofranil] Amitriptyline [Elavil] Clomipramine [Anafranil] a. Secondary amine tricyclics Nortriptyline [Pamelor] Desipramine [Norpramin] Protriptyline [Vivactil] b. Tetracyclics Maprotiline [Ludiomil] Amoxapine [Ascendin] c. Atypical tetracyclic Mirtazapine [Remeron]	Drowsiness,‡ headache,† dizziness usually due to orthostatic hypotension, excitation, anxiety, confusion in the elderly, seizures, EEG changes, tremor, extrapyramidal symptoms [rare], myoclonic twitches	Photosensitivity, vasculitis, erythema, urticaria, fever, pruritus, diaphoresis	Ventricular tachycardia; palpitations; hypertension; orthostatic hypotension; prolongation of the PR, QT, and QRS intervals; suppressed ST segment; flattened T wave	Dry mouth,‡ constipation,‡ urinary retention, adynamic ileus, abdominal pain or cramps, nausea/vomiting, anorexia, diarrhea, jaundice, weight gain 34.5%, altered glucose metabolism	SIADH	Agranulocytosis, eosinophilia, purpura, thrombocytopenia, leukopenia	Blurred vision,‡ mydriasis, increased intraocular pressure can precipitate crisis in patients with angle-closure glaucoma	Decreased libido, testicular swelling, painful or delayed ejaculation, delayed orgasm, breast enlargement, breast enlargement, galactorrhea (females), gynecomastia (males)
	Sedation† increased with lower doses, fatigue, dizziness, headache		Orthostatic hypotension	Dry mouth, constipation, increased appetite, weight gain average 6 kg		Agranulocytosis [rare], neutropenia [rare]	Blurred vision	

Table continued on following page

ANTIDEPRESSANT MEDICATIONS *Continued*

Adverse Effects

Chemical Class and Drug	Neurologic	Dermatologic	Cardiovascular	Digestive	Endocrine	Hematologic	Ocular	Other
4. Monocyclics Bupropion (Wellbutrin)	Increased risk of seizure at higher doses (bulimics at higher risk); 0.5% of patients receiving <450 mg/day, 2.2% of those receiving >450 mg/day; agitation, † insomnia†; anxiety; restlessness	Excessive diaphoresis, † pruritus, maculopapular rash	Hypertension 4.3%, dizziness, syncope 1.2%, palpitations, ventricular tachycardia, premature ventricular contractions	Dry mouth, ‡ constipation, † nausea/vomiting, † weight loss >5 pounds 28%, weight gain 9.4%, dysgeusia			Blurred vision 14.6%	Menstrual irregularity
5. Monoamine oxidase inhibitors (MAOIs) Phenelzine (Nardil) Tranylcypromine (Parnate)	Dizziness, † headache, † drowsiness, confusion, shaking, tremor; weakness, myoclonus, hyperreflexia, twitching, fatigue, insomnia*	Photophobia, diaphoresis	Hypertensive crisis most serious; tyramine-free diet required, palpitations, † orthostatic hypotension,† angina, peripheral edema*	Dry mouth, † constipation, † appetite stimulation and weight gain, † nausea/vomiting,* elevated hepatic enzymes, necrotizing hepatocellular damage (rare)		Rare: anemia, leukopenia, agranulocytosis, thrombocytopenia	Blurred vision, mydriasis	Fever, urinary retention, sexual dysfunction,† orgasm dysfunction, anorgasmia or delayed orgasm, ejaculation dysfunction, retarded or no ejaculation, priapism, impotence

6. Phenyl piperazines								
Nefazodone (Serzone)	Sedation,† memory impairment, paresthesias, abnormal dreams, decreased concentration, ataxia, incoordination, psychomotor impairment, tremor, hypertonia, headache, dizziness, insomnia	Flushing, pruritus, rash	Bradycardia, orthostatic hypotension	Dry mouth,† nausea/vomiting,* constipation,* dysgeusia	Polydipsia		Blurred vision, scotomata	Urinary urgency, urinary retention, vaginitis, breast pain, flu-like symptoms, fever, chills, neck rigidity, peripheral edema, arthralgia, increased coughing, tinnitus
Trazodone (Desyrel)	Sedation,† headache,† lightheadedness, nervousness, fatigue, muscle tremor, musculoskeletal pain		Hypotension, orthostatic hypotension, cardiac arrhythmias, ventricular tachycardia, various ECG changes	Dry mouth,† nausea*/vomiting		Neutropenia		Priapism, ejaculation dysfunction, retrograde or no ejaculation, orgasm dysfunction, anorgasmia, libido increase

*Less common.
†More common.
‡Very common.
ECG = electrocardiogram; EEG = electroencephalogram; SIADH = syndrome of inappropriate antidiuretic hormone.

ANTIPSYCHOTIC MEDICATIONS

Adverse Effects

Chemical Class and Drug	Neurologic	Dermatologic	Cardiovascular	Digestive	Endocrine	Hematologic	Ocular	Other
1. Phenothiazines								
a. Aliphatics								
Chlorpromazine (Thorazine)	Acute dystonia,* drug-induced parkinsonism,* akathisia, NMS, TD, seizures,† sedation, anticholinergic§	Photosensitivity, blue-gray discoloration of skin, allergic maculopapular rash first 2 months	Postural hypotension, prolongs QT and PR intervals, blunts T waves, depresses ST segment	Cholestatic jaundice* (look for itchiness, RUQ discomfort, nausea, fever, malaise)	Hyperprolactinemia: *females:* galactorrhea, amenorrhea; *males:* galactorrhea, impotence. Hyperthermia, weight gain	Agranulocytosis (rare)	Pigmentation, granular deposits of lens and cornea	Anorgasmia, decreased libido
b. Piperidines								
Thioridazine (Mellaril)	Acute dystonia,* drug-induced parkinsonism,* akathisia, NMS, TD, seizures,† sedation,* anticholinergic§	Photosensitivity	Slowed cardiac conduction, heart block, prolonged QT interval, postural hypotension		Hyperprolactinemia, hyperthermia, weight gain	Agranulocytosis (rare)	Pigmentation, pigmentary retinopathy (>800 mg/day)	Anorgasmia, decreased libido, retrograde ejaculation
Mesoridazine (Serentil)	Acute dystonia,* drug-induced parkinsonism,* akathisia,* NMS, TD, seizures, sedation, anticholinergic§	Photosensitivity	Slowed cardiac conduction, heart block, prolonged QT interval, postural hypotension		Hyperprolactinemia, hyperthermia, weight gain	Agranulocytosis (rare)	Pigmentation	Anorgasmia, decreased libido
c. Piperazines								
Fluphenazine (Prolixin)	Acute dystonia,‡ drug-induced parkinsonism,‡ akathisia,‡ NMS, TD, seizures,* sedation*		Orthostatic hypotension*		Hyperprolactinemia, hyperthermia, weight gain			Anorgasmia, decreased libido

Perphenazine (Trilafon)	Acute dystonia,† drug-induced parkinsonism,† akathisia,† NMS, TD, seizures, sedation*	Orthostatic hypotension†	Hyperprolactinemia, hyperthermia, weight gain	Anorgasmia, decreased libido
Trifluoperazine (Stelazine)	Acute dystonia,† drug-induced parkinsonism,‡ akathisia,‡ anticholinergic,§ NMS, TD, seizures, sedation*	Orthostatic hypotension†	Hyperprolactinemia, hyperthermia, weight gain	Anorgasmia, decreased libido
2. Thioxanthene Thiothixene (Navane)	Acute dystonia,‡ drug-induced parkinsonism,‡ akathisia,‡ NMS, TD, seizures, sedation*	Orthostatic hypotension*	Hyperprolactinemia, hyperthermia, weight gain	Ocular changes, pigmentation / Anorgasmia, decreased libido
3. Butyrophenones Haloperidol (Haldol)	Acute dystonia,‡ drug-induced parkinsonism,‡ akathisia,‡ NMS, TD, seizures,* sedation*	Orthostatic hypotension*	Hyperprolactinemia, hyperthermia, weight gain	Anorgasmia, decreased libido
4. Dihydroindolone Molindone (Moban)	Acute dystonia, drug-induced parkinsonism, akathisia, NMS, TD, seizures,* sedation*	Orthostatic hypotension*	Hyperprolactinemia,* hyperthermia, weight gain*	Anorgasmia, decreased libido

Table continued on following page

ANTIPSYCHOTIC MEDICATIONS *Continued*

Chemical Class and Drug	Adverse Effects						
	Neurologic	Dermatologic	Cardiovascular	Digestive	Endocrine	Hematologic	Ocular	Other

Chemical Class and Drug	Neurologic	Dermatologic	Cardiovascular	Digestive	Endocrine	Hematologic	Ocular	Other
5. Dibenzodiazepines								
Loxapine [Loxitane]	Acute dystonia, drug-induced parkinsonism, akathisia, NMS, TD, seizures,† sedation				Hyperprolactinemia, hyperthermia, weight gain			Anorgasmia, decreased libido
6. Diphenylbutylpiperidines								
Pimozide [Orap]	Acute dystonia, drug-induced parkinsonism, akathisia, NMS, TD, seizures, sedation				Hyperprolactinemia, hyperthermia, weight gain			Anorgasmia, decreased libido
7. Atypicals								
Clozapine [Clozaril]	Acute dystonia,* drug-induced parkinsonism,* akathisia.* NMS not documented with Clozapine alone, no TD, seizures† (dosage-dependent), sedation,† anticholinergic‡§		Tachycardia, postural hypotension,† dizziness, myoclonus	GI upset, constipation	Hyperprolactinemia, hyperthermia, weight gain	Agranulocytosis [1–3%], clinically insignificant leukocytosis, leukopenia, eosinophilia, increased ESR		Anorgasmia, decreased libido, sialorrhea, periodic catalepsy

Drug								
Risperidone (Risperdal)	Dose-related acute dystonia, dose-related drug-induced parkinsonism, dose-related akathisia, NMS, TD, sedation, anxiety, insomnia, seizures (especially with hyponatremia), decreased concentration	Rash	Prolonged QTc interval, postural hypotension, dizziness, tachycardia	Nausea, constipation, dyspepsia	Hyperprolactinemia, hyperthermia, weight gain	Thrombotic, thrombocytopenic purpura	Accommodation disturbances	Anorgasmia, decreased libido, rhinitis, priapism
Olanzapine (Zyprexa)	Agitation, nervousness, headache, insomnia, anxiety, somnolence, dizziness, akathisia*		Orthostatic hypotension	Liver enzyme elevation, dyspepsia, constipation, dry mouth	Weight gain, case reports of drug-induced diabetes/diabetic ketoacidosis			
Quetiapine (Seroquel)	Mild somnolence, syncope 1%; low risk for EPS, TD, NMS		Orthostatic hypotension	Elevated liver enzymes, dry mouth, constipation	Weight gain,* hypothyroidism		Cataracts in animal studies; ophthalmologic examination recommended before and every 6 months after treatment	Anorgasmia, decreased libido

*Less common.
†More common.
‡Very common.
§Anticholinergic side effects include dry mouth, constipation (possibly fecal impaction), blurred vision, delayed micturition (possibly urinary retention), narrow-angle glaucoma, and delirium.

EPS = Extrapyramidal side effects; GI = gastrointestinal; NMS = neuroleptic malignant syndrome; RUQ = right upper quadrant; TD = tardive dyskinesia.

MOOD-STABILIZING MEDICATIONS

Chemical Class and Drug	Adverse Effects							
	Neurologic	Dermatologic	Cardiovascular	Digestive	Endocrine	Hematologic	Renal	Other
1. Lithium	Tremor, fatigue, cognitive impairment, headache, syncope	Psoriasis, alopecia, acneiform eruptions, follicular and maculopapular eruptions	T-wave flattening or inversions, sinus dysrhythmia	GI distress, nausea, vomiting, decreased appetite	Thyroid disturbances, clinical hypothyroidism 5%	Benign leukocytosis	Polyuria and polydipsia, minimal-change glomerulonephritis (rare), interstitial nephritis (rare), renal failure	Weight gain, edema, risk of Ebstein's anomaly in fetus <0.1%
2. Valproic acid (Depakote)	Sedation, ataxia, dysarthria, tremor, dizziness, diplopia	Hair loss 5–10%, maculopapular rash		Fatal hepatotoxicity (rare), asymptomatic elevated LFTs, pancreatitis (rare), nausea, vomiting		Thrombocytopenia, platelet dysfunction		Weight gain, edema, fetal neural tube defects 3–6%, craniofacial and heart abnormalities (rare)

244

3. Carbamazepine (Tegretol)	Drowsiness, confusion, ataxia, hyperreflexia, clonus, tremor, dizziness, diplopia, dysarthria	Exfoliative dermatitis, erythema multiforme, Stevens-Johnson syndrome, toxic epidermal necrolysis [all rare]; benign pruritic rash 10–15% in first few weeks	Decreased cardiac conduction	Hepatitis, nausea, vomiting, constipation, diarrhea, anorexia, pancreatitis	SIADH	Benign leukocytopenia, agranulocytosis, pancytopenia, aplastic anemia	Lenticular opacities; use with caution in glaucoma, prostatic hypertrophy, diabetes, alcohol abuse; fetal neural tube defects 1%, craniofacial abnormalities, microcephaly, growth retardation
4. Gabapentin (Neurontin)	Somnolence, fatigue, ataxia, dizziness, diplopia, nystagmus, tremor, blurred vision		Hypertension	Increased or decreased appetite, dyspepsia, flatulence		Easy bruising	Gingivitis, arthralgia
5. Lamotrigine (Lamictal)	Dizziness, headache, diplopia, ataxia, somnolence	Rash 10%, Stevens-Johnson syndrome		GI upset, nausea, vomiting			Weight gain
6. Tiagabine	Dizziness						
7. Topiramate (Topamax)	Dizziness, sedation					Renal calculi	Weight loss

GI = gastrointestinal; LFT = liver function test; SIADH = syndrome of inappropriate antidiuretic hormone.

OTHER DRUGS

Adverse Effects

Chemical Class and Drug	Neurologic	Dermatologic	Cardiovascular	Endocrine	Digestive	Other
1. Adrenergic receptor blockers Propranolol [Inderal]	Depression, insomnia, fatigue, agitation,* confusion,* hallucinations*		Worsens AV conduction defects; complete AV heart block; hypotension,† bradycardia,† dizziness	Elevated blood glucose; can mask signs of hypoglycemia	Nausea, vomiting, diarrhea, constipation, abdominal discomfort	Relatively contraindicated in patients with COPD, bronchial asthma, diabetes, CHF, persistent angina, or peripheral vascular disease; use with caution in patients with renal or hepatic disease; sexual dysfunction
2. Dopamine agonist Amantadine [Symmetrel]	Mild dizziness, insomnia, impaired concentration, irritability,* depression,* anxiety,* dysarthria,* ataxia,* seizures, psychotic signs and symptoms, headache	Blotchy spots on skin			Nausea, anorexia	Relatively contraindicated in patients with renal abnormality or seizure disorder; use cautiously in patients with edema or cardiovascular disease
3. Anticholinergics Benztropine [Cogentin] Trihexyphenidyl hydrochloride [Artane]	Delirium, memory impairment		Sinus tachycardia		Constipation, decreased salivation	Blurred vision, narrow-angle glaucoma, photophobia, decreased sweating, hyperthermia, delayed or retrograde ejaculation, worsened asthma, urinary retention
4. Antihistamines Diphenhydramine [Benadryl]	Sedation, dizziness, poor motor coordination, dry mouth, urinary retention		Hypotension		Epigastric discomfort, nausea, vomiting, diarrhea, constipation	Blurred vision; use cautiously in patients with urinary problems, asthma, enlarged prostate, or glaucoma

Drug	CNS/Neurologic effects	Dermatologic	Cardiovascular	GI/Hepatic	Other
5. Benzodiazepines	Drowsiness, dizziness, ataxia, disinhibition, cognitive deficits,* anterograde amnesia, paradoxical aggression	Maculopapular rash*		Increased toxicity in hepatically impaired	Withdrawal signs and symptoms: anxiety, insomnia, headache, nausea, tremor; sweating, dizziness, increased sensory perception, decreased concentration, respiratory depression, increased aggression in brain damage; use in pregnancy associated with cleft palate; use with caution in renal diagnosis [dx]; cognitive dx, hepatic dx, porphyria, myasthenia gravis
6. Buspirone [Buspar]	Dizziness, headache, excitement, nervousness, light-headedness, insomnia				
7. Zolpidem [Ambien]	Dizziness, morning hangover; anterograde amnesia			Nausea	
8. Zaleplon [Sonata]	Sedation, dizziness			GI upset, nausea, vomiting	
9. Psychostimulants Dextroamphetamine [Dexedrine] Methylphenidate [Ritalin] Pemoline [Cylert]	Psychomotor agitation, insomnia, dizziness, tremor; euphoria, precipitation of tics, Tourette's syndrome, headache with pemoline only; choreiform movements, dyskinesia, night terrors, lip licking or biting	Hypersensitivity rash, hives, conjunctivitis	Palpitations, tachycardia, hypertension	Anorexia, dry mouth, weight loss, diarrhea, constipation with pemoline only: chemical hepatitis	Growth delay in children, depression, psychosis [rare]

Table continued on following page

OTHER DRUGS *Continued*

Chemical Class and Drug	Adverse Effects					
	Neurologic	Dermatologic	Cardiovascular	Endocrine	Digestive	Other
10. Substance dependence						
Clonidine [Catapres]	Sedation, dizziness, fatigue, insomnia	Photophobia, rash	Hypotension		Weight gain, dry mouth, nausea, constipation	Sexual dysfunction, anxiety, depression
Disulfiram [Antabuse]	Sedation, fatigue, headache, peripheral neuropathy (rare), optic neuritis (rare), irritability, psychosis (rare)	Acne, rash			Hepatotoxicity, metallic aftertaste	Impotence
Methadone [Dolophine]	Sedation, dizziness				Nausea, emesis, constipation, dry mouth	Tolerance along with physiologic and psychologic dependence, depression, urinary retention, euphoria or dysphoria, diaphoresis
Naltrexone [ReVia]	Insomnia, headache, dizziness				Hepatocellular injury at high doses, nausea, weight loss	May precipitate acute opiate withdrawal in patients using opiates; fatigue, anxiety, joint and muscle pain

*Less common.
†More common.
AV = atrioventricular; CHF = congestive heart failure; COPD = chronic obstructive pulmonary disease.

APPENDIX L

Physical and Behavioral Indicators of Abuse

MARK KRUSHELNYCKY
AVA ALBRECHT

Type of Abuse	Physical Indicators	Behavioral Indicators
Physical abuse	*Unexplained bruises and welts:* on face, lips, mouth, torso, back, buttocks or thighs, clustered in various stages of healing; forming regular patterns like articles used to inflict wounds (electric cord, belt buckle); on several surface areas; regularly after absence from school or work, weekend, or vacation *Unexplained burns:* cigar or cigarette burns, especially on soles, palms, back, or buttocks; immersion burns (sock-like, glove-like, doughnut-shaped on buttocks or genitalia); patterned like electric burner, iron; rope burns on arms, legs, neck, torso; infected burns, indicating delay in seeking treatment *Unexplained fractures or dislocations* to skull, nose, or facial structure in various stages of healing; multiple or spinal fractures *Unexplained lacerations* to mouth, lips, gums, eyes, or external genitalia in various stages of healing; bald patches on scalp	Feels deserving of punishment; wary of adult contacts; apprehensive when other children cry. Behavioral extremes: aggressiveness or withdrawal. Frightened of parents, afraid to go home, reports injury by parents. Vacant or frozen stare; lies very still while surveying surroundings; does not cry when approached by examiner; responds to questions in monosyllables. Inappropriate or precocious maturity; manipulative behavior to get attention. Capable of only superficial relationships. Indiscriminately seeks affection; poor self-concept
Physical neglect	Underweight, poor growth pattern, failure to thrive. Consistent hunger, poor hygiene, inappropriate dress. Consistent lack of supervision, especially during dangerous activities or for long periods. Wasting of subcutaneous tissue; unattended physical problems or medical needs; abandonment. Abdominal distension; bald patches on the scalp	Begging, stealing food; extended stays at school (early arrival and late departure); rare attendance at school; constant fatigue, listlessness, or falling asleep in class. Inappropriate seeking of affection; assuming adult responsibilities and concerns. Alcohol or drug abuse; delinquency (thefts); states there is no caretaker

Sexual abuse	Difficulty in walking or sitting; torn, stained, or bloody underclothing; pain, swelling, or itching in genital area; pain on urination; bruises, bleeding, or lacerations in external genitalia or vaginal or anal areas; vaginal or penile discharge; venereal disease, especially in preteens; poor sphincter tone; pregnancy	Unwilling to change for gym or participate in physical education class; withdrawal, fantasy, or infantile behavior or knowledge; poor peer relationships; delinquent or runaway; reports sexual assault by caretaker. Change in performance in school; suicidal behavior; sexual promiscuity
Emotional maltreatment	Speech disorders; lag in physical development; failure to thrive; hyperactive or disruptive behavior	Habit disorders (sucking, biting, rocking); conduct or learning disorders (antisocial, destructive); neurotic traits (sleep disorders, inhibition of play, unusual fearfulness); psychoneurotic reactions (hysteria, obsessions, compulsions, phobias, hypochondria). Behavior extremes (compliant, passive; aggressive, demanding); overly adaptive behavior (inappropriately adult, inappropriately infantile); developmental lags (mental, emotional); attempted suicide

From Lauer JW, Laurie IS, Salus MK, et al: The Role of the Mental Health Professional in the Prevention and Treatment of Child Abuse and Neglect. Washington, DC, U.S. Department of Health, Education and Welfare, National Center on Child Abuse and Neglect, 1979.

APPENDIX M
Elder Abuse and Neglect

CERI E. HADDA

Elder abuse and neglect have been estimated to occur in 10% of people older than 65 years of age. Abuse can be roughly divided into categories of physical, sexual, and psychologic abuse or neglect; financial exploitation; and self-abuse, self-neglect, and abandonment.

Remember

Be wary of caregivers who do not allow a patient to be examined or interviewed out of their presence.

Even a demented patient may be capable of expressing signs of abuse or neglect.

Elders at high risk for abuse and neglect include those with a functional, medical, or cognitive disability and those whose disability is worsening, leading to increased caregiver stress.

The highest proportion of elder abusers are adult children of elderly parents. Spouses, grandchildren, paid caregivers, staff, and visitors to other patients in a hospital or institutional setting should also be considered when abuse is suspected.

Caregivers with emotional, psychiatric, financial, or substance abuse problems are at higher risk to commit elder abuse or neglect, especially when the caregiver is an adult child who is dependent on the elderly parent.

The on-call physician is most likely to encounter the following signs and symptoms of abuse and neglect, either at the bedside or in the emergency room.

Physical Abuse

Physical abuse involves force leading to bodily injury, pain, or physical impairment, including
- Obvious acts of violence
- Physical punishment
- Inappropriate use of physical or chemical restraints
- Inappropriate use or withholding of medications
- Force feeding or withholding of nutrients or fluids

Signs and symptoms include
- Bruises
- Burns
- Lacerations
- Bone fractures
- Untreated injuries at different stages of healing

- Laboratory findings consistent with dehydration
- Excessive or inappropriately low use of medication
- Sudden change in behavior
- Report by the patient of being mistreated
- Refusal by the caregiver to allow access to the patient

Sexual Abuse

Sexual abuse involves any nonconsensual sexual contact, including contact involving an individual who is not competent to provide consent to such contact.

Signs and symptoms include
- Bruising or bite marks on the breasts, genitals, or buttocks
- Unexplained vaginal/anal bleeding or lacerations
- Unexplained venereal or genital infections
- Report by the patient of being sexually assaulted

Emotional Abuse

Emotional abuse involves infliction of emotional pain or distress via verbal or nonverbal acts. This can include verbal abuse, intimidation or humiliation, harassment, and isolating the patient via enforced social isolation or verbal withdrawal.

Signs and symptoms include
- Emotional lability or agitation
- Flat, withdrawn affect
- Regressive behaviors, including rocking and sucking
- Hypervigilance or excessive fearfulness

Neglect

Neglect involves either intentional or inadvertent failure to provide necessary care for an elder, including failing to provide food, clothing, shelter, and medication as well as a clean body and clothing and an appropriate living environment. This may involve either a service provider such as a home attendant or a family member.

Signs and symptoms include
- Dehydration or malnourishment
- Poor personal hygiene
- Untreated health problems such as bed sores
- Urine, feces, and/or dirt on patient and/or patient's clothing
- Attire that is inappropriate for the season
- Evidence or a patient's report of inadequate living conditions, including lack of heat, air conditioning, and running water

Self-Neglect and Self-Abuse

Self-neglect and self-abuse refer to the inability of an elderly person to maintain adequate self-care, jeopardizing his or her health or safety. The signs and symptoms parallel those for neglect or abuse by someone other than the elder. In this situation, homelessness or a severely inadequate or dangerous living arrangement may also be considered an indicator of self-neglect or self-abuse.

As with other situations involving assessment of danger to self, however, the person being evaluated **must** be deemed mentally incompetent in order to be legally regarded as self-neglecting or self-abusive. Nonetheless, if you are concerned about a patient, you should strongly consider encouraging the patient to accept additional consultations, for example, from a social worker or substance abuse counselor.

Abandonment

An elderly person is considered abandoned if he or she has been deserted by someone—either a family member or other caregiver—who was previously providing essential care. Frequent sites for abandonment include emergency rooms, public areas such as parks or stores, hospitals, and nursing facilities.

If You Suspect Elder Abuse or Neglect

Elder abuse is currently defined by state laws, and these laws can vary widely. Nonetheless, most states have mandatory laws regarding reporting even suspected abuse. All 50 states and the District of Columbia have some type of adult protective services (APS) to facilitate the reporting, investigating, and reduction of elder abuse. For persons working in a hospital setting, the social work department can usually provide assistance in reporting potential abuse as well as determining what, if anything, needs to be done to ensure safety for those at risk. As with child abuse, when elder abuse is suspected, the safety of the patient is primary.

For a referral to a state agency if abuse and/or neglect is suspected: Call National Eldercare Locator at 1-800-677-1116.

To locate an adult protection service (for domestic abuse/neglect) or an ombudsmen (for nursing home and other institutional abuse) in any state: Log on to www.elderabusecenter.org

APPENDIX N
Important Telephone Numbers

ERWIN C. TING

Only nationwide telephone numbers in the United States are listed below. Consult your local telephone book for local numbers.

AIDS

AIDS Hotline
1-800-342-2437

Alcoholism

Abuse of Alcohol 24-Hour Helpline and Treatment
1-800-222-0469

Alzheimer's Disease

Alzheimer's Disease and Related Disorders Association
1-800-272-3900

Children's and Family Services

Child Abuse and Neglect Information Prevention Resource Center
1-800-342-7472

Child Abuse Hotline
1-800-422-4453

Parents Anonymous
1-800-231-0353

Crisis Intervention

National Runaway Switchboard
1-800-621-4000

Domestic Violence Hotline
1-800-942-6906

Drug Abuse and Other Addictive Behaviors

Drug Helpline
1-800-378-4435

800 Cocaine Information
1-800-262-2463

Focus on Recovery Helpline
1-800-234-0420
1-800-234-0246

National Council on Compulsive Gambling
1-800-522-4700

Epilepsy

Epilepsy Foundation of America
1-800-332-1000

Suicide

NAMI Helpline
1-800-950-NAMI

American Association of Suicidology
202-237-2280
1-800-SUICIDE

On Call Formulary

HILLERY BOSWORTH
PATRICK YING

The On Call Formulary is a quick reference for information on medications that are commonly encountered while on call. Doses listed are for adults with normal renal and hepatic function unless otherwise noted, and generic names are listed. For further information, consult your pharmacy or the medication insert instructions.

Acetaminophen (Tylenol)   *Analgesic, antipyretic*

Indications:	Pain, fever.
Actions:	Raises the pain threshold; acts directly on the hypothalamic heat-regulating center.
Side effects:	Uncommon—rash, drug fever, mucosal ulcerations, leukopenia, and pancytopenia.
Comments:	Unlike aspirin, acetaminophen has no anti-inflammatory action, does not irritate the stomach, does not affect the aggregation of platelets, and does not interact with oral anticoagulants. It is hepatotoxic in overdose; use carefully in patients with liver disease.
Dose:	325 to 1000 mg PO every 4 to 6 hours PRN up to 4000 mg daily.

Adderall (see **Dextroamphetamine/Amphetamine**)

Alprazolam (Xanax)   *Benzodiazepine*

Indications:	Anxiety, tension.
Actions:	Depresses the CNS at the limbic and subcortical levels. Produces an anxiolytic effect by enhancing the effect of the neurotransmitter gamma-aminobutyric acid (GABA), which increases inhibition and blocks cortical and limbic arousal.
Side effects:	Confusion, drowsiness, ataxia, tremor, hypotension, bradycardia, blurred vision, constipation, nausea, vomiting, and respiratory depression. Use with care in patients with respiratory compromise, such as COPD.
Comments:	Alprazolam is one of the more potent and short-acting of the benzodiazepines. Associated with inter-dose anxiety and higher risk of dependence because of its rapid onset of action. Lower doses are effective in elderly patients and in patients with renal or hepatic dysfunction.

Dose: Usual starting dose is 0.25 to 0.5 mg PO TID. Can increase up to 1 mg/day in divided doses every 3 to 4 days. In elderly or debilitated patients, usual starting dose is 0.25 mg BID or TID.

Aluminum hydroxide–magnesium hydroxide (see Maalox)

Amantadine (Symmetrel)   *Antiparkinsonian agent*

Indications: Drug-induced extrapyramidal reactions, idiopathic parkinsonism, parkinsonian syndrome.
Actions: Thought to cause the release of dopamine in the substantia nigra.
Side effects: Confusion, anxiety, psychosis, ataxia, insomnia, orthostatic hypotension, CHF, nausea, vomiting, and urine retention.
Comments: Use cautiously in patients with a history of hepatic disease, seizures, psychosis, renal disease, and CHF. Less commonly used than anticholinergic agents for drug-induced parkinsonism.
Dose: 100 mg BID or TID.

Ambien (see Zolpidem)

Amitriptyline (Elavil)   *Tricyclic antidepressant*

Indications: Depression, chronic pain syndromes.
Actions: Inhibits presynaptic reuptake of norepinephrine, serotonin, and dopamine.
Side effects: High in sedating, anticholinergic, and orthostatic hypotensive effects. Other effects include sedation, confusion, seizures, orthostatic hypotension, tachycardia, arrhythmias, MI, heart block, CHF, ECG changes, blurred vision, dry mouth, constipation, nausea, vomiting, glaucoma exacerbation, and urinary retention.
Interactions: Contraindicated within 2 weeks of MAOI. Potentiates anticholinergic effects of other medications.
Comments: Abrupt withdrawal of long-term therapy can cause nausea, headache, and malaise. If signs of hypersensitivity occur, drug should be tapered and discontinued. Has a high incidence of sedation, but tolerance to this effect usually develops after several weeks.
Dose: 50 to 100 mg daily divided TID. Increase to 200 mg daily. Maximum dosage is 300 mg daily.

Antabuse (see Disulfiram)

Aricept (see Donepezil)

Ativan (see Lorazepam)

Benztropine (Cogentin)   *Anticholinergic, antiparkinsonian agent*

Indications: Acute dystonia, antipsychotic drug–induced parkinsonism, akathisia.
Actions: Has anticholinergic and antihistaminic activity.

Side effects:	Has anticholinergic and antihistaminic side effects, including disorientation, agitation, confusion, psychosis, delirium, palpitations, blurred vision, dilated pupils, dry mouth, nausea, vomiting, constipation, and urinary retention.
Comments:	Use cautiously in elderly patients because of CNS effects. Anticholinergics are the second choice for treating akathisia, after beta-adrenergic blockers.
Dose:	For acute dystonia, 2 mg IM or IV. If no effect in 20 minutes, repeat the injection. If there is still no effect, a benzodiazepine, such as lorazepam 1 mg IM or IV, can be tried. Follow with benztropine 1 to 2 mg PO BID to prevent recurrence. For drug-induced parkinsonism, 1 to 2 mg PO BID (reduce doses in elderly patients). For akathisia, 2 mg PO BID.

Bromocriptine   *Dopamine antagonist, antiparkinsonian agent*
(Parlodel)

Indications:	Parkinson's disease.
Actions:	Activates dopaminergic receptors in the neostriatum of the CNS.
Side effects:	Most are mild to moderate, with nausea being the most common. Others include mania, delusions, insomnia, hypotension, nausea, and vomiting.
Comments:	May potentiate antihypertensive agents. Bromocriptine is usually given with either levodopa alone or levodopa-carbidopa combination.
Dose:	Initial dose of 1.25 mg PO BID with meals. May be increased every 14 to 28 days up to 100 mg daily or until maximum therapeutic response is achieved (therapeutic range is usually from 2.5 to 15 mg/day).

Bupropion (Wellbutrin;   *Antidepressant*
sustained release:
Wellbutrin SR, Zyban)

Indications:	Depression. Sustained release form indicated for smoking cessation.
Actions:	Mechanism of action is unknown. It is a weak inhibitor of norepinephrine, dopamine, and serotonin reuptake.
Side effects:	Akathisia, anxiety, confusion, decreased libido, insomnia, sedation, arrhythmias, blurred vision, nausea, vomiting, and dry mouth.
Interactions:	Cimetidine increases bupropion levels.
Comments:	Doses greater than 450 mg daily have been associated with seizures. Contraindicated in patients who have taken MAOIs in the previous 14 days and in those with seizure or eating disorders.
Dose:	For slow release (SR), 150 mg PO every morning for 3 days, increase up to 200 mg BID. For immediate release, initially 100 mg PO BID. Increase after 3 days to usual dosage of 100 mg TID. If no response after several weeks, consider increasing to 150 mg TID. To reduce the seizure risk, patients should not receive

more than 150 mg in a single dose or more than 450 mg daily. If used for smoking cessation, do not use doses over 300 mg per day.

BuSpar (see Buspirone)

Buspirone (BuSpar) *Anxiolytic*

Indications: Anxiety, SSRI augmentation.
Actions: Precise mechanism of action is unknown. Not related to benzodiazepines, barbiturates, or other sedatives and anxiolytics. Appears to affect several neurotransmitters, including serotonin, norepinephrine, and GABA.
Side effects: Dizziness, drowsiness, insomnia, palpitations, blurred vision, nausea, dry mouth, constipation, and diarrhea.
Comments: Use cautiously in patients with impaired hepatic or renal function. May displace digoxin from serum-binding sites when the two drugs are used together.
Dose: Initially 5 mg PO TID. May be increased at 3-day intervals by 5 mg/day. Usual dose is 20 to 30 mg daily in divided doses; maximum dose 60 mg/day.

Carbamazepine (Tegretol) *Anticonvulsant*

Indications: Seizure disorder, bipolar disorder.
Actions: Mechanism of action is unknown.
Side effects: Dizziness, ataxia, sedation, dysarthria, diplopia, nausea and GI upset, reversible mild leukopenia, and reversible increase in LFTs. Less common: SIADH, cardiac conduction delay, tremor, memory disturbance, and confusional states. Idiosyncratic and severe: hepatitis, aplastic anemia, thrombocytopenia, and leukopenia.
Comments: Before initiation, must perform CBC and LFTs. Therapeutic levels are 4 to 12 μg/mL. May be more effective than lithium for rapid cycling bipolar disorder. Induces microsomal enzymes, which will lower levels of many drugs including itself. Serum levels should be monitored frequently for first few months. CBC should be monitored regularly or if signs of infection or blood abnormality occur. Drug should be stopped if WBC <3000/mm^3, ANC <1500/mm^3, or platelets <100,000/mm^3.
Dose: Initially, 200 mg PO BID. May increase by 200 mg PO every 3 to 4 days in divided doses. Maintenance dosage may range from 600 to 1600 mg daily.

Catapres (see Clonidine)

Celexa (see Citalopram)

Chloral Hydrate (Noctec) *Sedative, hypnotic*

Indications: Sedation, insomnia, premedication for EEG, hypnosis.
Actions: Nonspecific CNS depressant similar to barbiturates.
Side effects: Nausea, vomiting, headache, ataxia, confusion, rash, dependence, liver toxicity, dependence.

Interactions:	With IV furosemide can cause BP instability and flushing.
Comments:	Not a first-line drug because of the potential for toxic effects. Monitor vital signs. Drug may displace oral anticoagulants, such as warfarin, from protein binding sites. Overdose may cause respiratory depression, coma, and death.
Dose:	500 to 1000 mg PO QHS. For children, 25 to 50 mg/kg.

Chlordiazepoxide (Librium) *Benzodiazepine*

Indications:	Alcohol withdrawal, anxiety, sedation.
Actions:	Depresses the CNS at the limbic and subcortical levels. Enhances the effect of the neurotransmitter GABA.
Side effects:	Confusion, sedation, ataxia, and respiratory depression. Use with care in patients with respiratory compromise, such as COPD. At high doses, paradoxical reaction of rage and disinhibition.
Comments:	Risk of dependence. Preferred use is for alcohol withdrawal rather than as a sedative-hypnotic owing to its long half-life.
Dose:	25 to 50 mg PO TID or QID for alcohol withdrawal. May increase to maximum dose of 300 mg daily.

Chlorpromazine (Thorazine) *Antipsychotic*

Indications:	Psychosis, agitation.
Actions:	Postsynaptic blockade of CNS dopamine receptors.
Side effects:	Orthostatic hypotension, dry mouth, constipation, dizziness, drowsiness, and retrograde ejaculation. EPS, tardive dyskinesia, dystonic reactions possible.
Comments:	Low-potency antipsychotic. More likely to cause sedation, hypotension, anticholinergic, and dermatologic side effects than other antipsychotics. Also has highest risk for seizures and agranulocytosis compared with other typical antipsychotics.
Dose:	Start at 50 to 100 mg PO TID or QID; titrate up 100 mg every 2 days to an effective dose, usually 300 to 800 mg. For acute agitation use 100 to 200 mg PO every 4 hours PRN or 25 to 50 mg IM every 4 hours PRN.

Citalopram (Celexa) *SSRI antidepressant*

Indications:	Depression.
Actions:	Blocks presynaptic serotonin reuptake.
Side effects:	Nausea, somnolence, sexual dysfunction.
Interactions:	Mildly increases TCA and antiarrhythmic levels. Contraindicated within 2 weeks of MAOI.
Comments:	Has the fewest known cytochrome interactions of the SSRIs.
Dose:	20 to 40 mg PO QD. Start with 10 mg QD in elderly. May titrate up to 60 mg QD after a 4 to 6 week trial.

Clomipramine (Anafranil)   *Tricyclic antidepressant*

Indications:	Obsessive-compulsive disorder.
Actions:	Blocks serotonin, norepinephrine, and dopamine reuptake.
Side effects:	Sedation, postural hypotension, sexual dysfunction, seizures, and anticholinergic effects, including dry mouth, blurred vision, constipation, and urinary retention.
Interactions:	Contraindicated within 2 weeks of MAOI. Levels may increase with some SSRIs.
Comments:	Treatment with clomipramine is limited by anticholinergic effects.
Dose:	Start 20 mg PO QHS; titrate to 150 to 250 mg PO daily.

Clonazepam (Klonopin)   *Benzodiazepine*

Indications:	Anxiety, panic disorder, anticonvulsant.
Actions:	Depresses the CNS at the limbic and subcortical levels. Enhances the effect of the neurotransmitter GABA.
Side effects:	Confusion, drowsiness, ataxia, tremor, hypotension, bradycardia, blurred vision, constipation, nausea, vomiting, and respiratory depression. Use with care in patients with respiratory compromise, such as COPD.
Comments:	Abrupt withdrawal may precipitate status epilepticus. Monitor CBC and LFTs periodically. May cause dependence. May be associated with the emergence of depression.
Dose:	For panic and anxiety, 0.5 to 6 mg daily usually divided in two to three doses.

Clonidine (Catapres)   *Antihypertensive*

Indications:	Opioid withdrawal, Tourette's syndrome, akathisia.
Actions:	Mechanism of action is as an agonist at alpha-adrenergic receptors.
Side effects:	Sedation, insomnia, nightmares, restlessness, anxiety, and depression. Hallucinations are rare.
Comments:	Overdose may cause decreased blood pressure, heart rate, and respiratory rate. Clonidine is begun at low doses to minimize side effects. Not the preferred treatment for akathisia.
Dose:	Start with initial dose as low as 0.05 mg daily, and increase slowly by no more than 0.1 mg daily until therapeutic effects are achieved. Usual daily dose is 0.1 to 0.3 mg in two to three divided doses. Clonidine should not be stopped abruptly. Taper off slowly to prevent rebound hypertension.

Clorazepate (Tranxene)   *Benzodiazepine*

Indications:	Generalized anxiety, alcohol withdrawal.
Actions:	Depresses the CNS at the limbic and subcortical levels. Enhances the effect of the neurotransmitter GABA.

Side effects:	Confusion, drowsiness, ataxia, tremor, hypotension, bradycardia, blurred vision, constipation, nausea, vomiting, and respiratory depression.
Comments:	Is metabolized into desmethyldiazepam by stomach acid.
Dose:	7.5 to 15 mg BID to QID; after stabilization of dose, can be given in a single dose formulation of 11.25 or 22.5 mg PO QHS.

Clozapine (Clozaril) *Atypical antipsychotic*

Indications:	Treatment-resistant schizophrenia.
Actions:	Thought to work mainly through blockade of D_1 and D_4 (dopamine) receptors and of 5-HT_2 (serotonin) receptors.
Side effects:	Agranulocytosis, seizures, postural hypotension, sedation, hypersalivation, tachycardia, constipation, transient hyperthermia, weight gain, and eosinophilia.
Comments:	Must obtain baseline CBC and monitor CBC weekly thereafter for decrease in granulocytes. If WBC >3000/mm^3 for the first 6 months, then can monitor CBC every other week. If WBC <3000/mm^3 or ANC <1500/mm^3, drug should be stopped and CBC should be checked daily. Can consider rechallenge if WBC >3000/mm^3 and ANC >1500/mm^3 and no signs of infection have occurred. At doses above 600 mg daily, risk of seizures increases greatly. Plasma concentrations may be increased by drugs that inhibit cytochrome P450, such as cimetidine and SSRIs.
Dose:	Begin with a single 25-mg dose and increase by no more than 25 mg daily to a daily dosage of 300 to 450 mg in divided doses. Doses should then be increased by no more than 100 mg once or twice a week. Titration should be slow to avoid hypotension, sedation, and seizures. Maximum daily dosage is 900 mg.

Clozaril (see Clozapine)

Cogentin (see Benztropine)

Cognex (see Tacrine)

Compazine (see Prochlorperazine)

Coumadin (see Warfarin)

Cylert (see Pemoline)

Dantrolene Sodium *Muscle relaxant*

Indications:	NMS, chronic spasticity.
Actions:	Dissociates the excitation-contraction coupling of skeletal muscle, probably interfering with the release of calcium from the sarcoplasmic reticulum.
Side effects:	Hepatotoxicity, drowsiness, dizziness, weakness, malaise, and diarrhea.

Comments: May decrease rigidity, hyperthermia, and tachycardia associated with NMS. Symptomatic hepatitis has been reported at various doses and can be fatal. Risk of hepatic injury is greater in females and persons older than 35 years.
Dose: 1 to 3 mg/kg IV every 6 hours to a maximum daily dose of 10 mg/kg and then 4 to 8 mg/kg/day PO divided into a QID regimen for NMS.

Depakene (see Valproic acid)

Depakote (see Valproic acid)

Desipramine (Norpramin)   *Tricyclic antidepressant*

Indications: Depression.
Actions: Inhibits epinephrine, dopamine, and serotonin reuptake.
Side effects: Sedation, postural hypotension, and anticholinergic effects. See Amitriptyline.
Interactions: Contraindicated within 2 weeks of MAOI. Levels may increase with some SSRIs.
Comments: Less sedating and fewer anticholinergic effects than most other tricyclics. ECGs and blood levels should be monitored. Therapeutic level is 125 to 300 ng/mL.
Dose: Start 20 mg PO QHS and titrate to 150 to 200 mg QD. Begin with low dose and titrate slowly. Doses range from 50 to 300 mg daily.

Desyrel (see Trazodone)

Dexedrine (see Dextroamphetamine)

Dextroamphetamine (Dexedrine)   *Psychostimulant*

Indications: Attention-deficit/hyperactivity disorder, narcolepsy.
Actions: Sympathomimetic amine, which causes release of norepinephrine, dopamine, and serotonin from CNS nerve terminals.
Side effects: Restlessness, tremor, insomnia, dysphoria, psychosis, tachycardia, hypertension, rash, nausea, and vomiting.
Comments: Prolonged use may lead to tolerance and dependence. May be used to augment antidepressants. Also used to treat apathy in the depressed medically ill patient.
Dose: 5 to 30 mg/day PO in divided doses. May increase to 60 mg/day. Avoid HS dosing.

Dextroamphetamine/Amphetamine (Adderall)   *Stimulant*

Indications: Attention-deficit disorder, narcolepsy.
Actions: Blocks reuptake of dopamine and norepinephrine from the synapse, inhibits action of monoamine oxidase.
Side effects: Tachycardia, palpitation hypertension, diarrhea, constipation, overstimulation, insomnia, restlessness, psychosis (rare).

Comments: May precipitate hypertensive crisis or serotonin syn-
              drome in patients receiving MAOIs. Wait 14 days after
              administration of last dose of MAOI; also avoid TCAs,
              as they may potentiate effects.
Dose: For children 6 years and older, start 5 mg PO QD or BID
              and increase at 5 mg/day at weekly intervals until
              clinical effect is desired. Rarely will doses >40 mg be
              needed. For children 3 to 6 years old, start at 2.5 mg
              QD and increase 2.5 mg/day at weekly intervals.

Diazepam (Valium)   *Benzodiazepine*

Indications: Anxiety, sedation, alcohol withdrawal.
Actions: Depresses the CNS at the limbic and subcortical levels.
               Enhances the effect of the neurotransmitter GABA.
Side effects: Confusion, sedation, ataxia, respiratory depression at
               high doses. Use with care in patients with respiratory
               compromise, such as COPD. Paradoxical reaction of
               rage and disinhibition.
Comments: May cause dependence with prolonged use. Rapidly ab-
               sorbed but has long half-life and active metabolites.
               Caution should be used in elderly and patients with
               liver disease. IV formulation available but IM not rec-
               ommended because of incomplete absorption.
Dose: 5 to 10 mg PO BID to QID.

Dilantin (see **Phenytoin**)

Diphenhydramine (Benadryl)   *Antihistamine*

Indications: Insomnia, acute dystonia, akathisia, drug-induced par-
               kinsonism.
Actions: Anticholinergic and antihistaminic activity.
Side effects: Sedation, dizziness, dry mouth, urinary retention,
               blurred vision, glaucoma exacerbation, and confusion
               in the elderly.
Interactions: Potentiates anticholinergic effects of other medications.
               Contraindicated within 2 weeks of MAOI.
Comments: Second-line treatment for akathisia and EPS.
Dose: For insomnia, 25 to 50 mg PO QHS. For akathisia and
               drug-induced parkinsonism, 25 to 50 mg PO BID. For
               acute dystonia, 50 mg IM. May repeat in 20 minutes
               if no response.

Disulfiram (Antabuse)   *Alcohol deterrent*

Indications: Alcohol abuse.
Actions: Inhibits aldehyde dehydrogenase.
Side effects: Fatigue, drowsiness, body odor, halitosis, tremor, head-
               ache, dizziness, impotence, and foul taste in mouth.
               May exacerbate psychosis in patients with psychotic
               disorders.
Comments: Also inhibits enzymes interfering with the metabolism
               of a variety of drugs, including phenytoin, isoniazid,

warfarin, rifampin, barbiturates, and long-acting benzodiazepines. Ingestion of alcohol, even in small
amounts, can produce flushing, throbbing headache,
nausea, vomiting, sweating, thirst, dyspnea, hyperven-
tilation, tachycardia, blurred vision, and confusion. In
severe cases, there may be respiratory depression, cardiovascular collapse, arrhythmias, myocardial infarction, unconsciousness, convulsions, and death.
Treatment of severe reaction is supportive. Should be
given at least 12 hours after last alcohol ingestion, and
reaction can occur 1 to 2 weeks after last dose of
disulfiram.

Dose: 250 to 500 mg PO QHS.

Donepezil (Aricept)   *Acetylcholinesterase inhibitor*

Indications: Treatment of cognitive impairment associated with early Alzheimer's disease.
Actions: Reversible selective acetylcholinesterase inhibitor.
Side effects: Nausea, diarrhea, vomiting, muscle cramps, fatigue, and anorexia.
Comments: Cognitive improvement is temporary; rate of decline may, however, be slower with treatment.
Dose: 5 mg PO QHS; may increase to 10 mg PO QHS after 4 weeks.

Doxepin (Sinequan)   *Tricyclic antidepressant*

Indication: Depression, insomnia, anxiety, chronic pain syndromes.
Actions: Inhibits reuptake of serotonin, dopamine, and epineph-rine.
Side effects: Orthostatic hypotension. Very sedating and high inci-dence of anticholinergic effects. See Amitriptyline.
Interactions: Contraindicated within 2 weeks of MAOI. Levels may increase with some SSRIs.
Dose: Start 25 mg PO QHS; titrate to 150 to 300 mg QD.

Droperidol (Inapsine)   *Antipsychotic*

Indications: Severe agitation.
Actions: Postsynaptic blockade of dopamine receptors.
Side effects: Acute dystonia, parkinsonism, akathisia, NMS, tardive dyskinesia with long-term use, QT prolongation on ECG, postural hypotension, blurred vision, hyperpro-lactinemia, exacerbation of glaucoma.
Comments: Very-high-potency antipsychotic. Approved for use as an anesthetic agent; is used in severe agitation because it is rapidly absorbed parenterally; peak effect within 30 minutes.
Dose: 2.5 to 5 mg IM every 30 to 60 minutes; total doses between 5 and 20 mg usually adequate.

Effexor (see **Venlafaxine**)

Eldepryl (see **Selegiline**)

Eskalith (see **Lithium carbonate**)

Flumazenil (Romazicon)   *Benzodiazepine antagonist*

Indications:	Reversal of benzodiazepine sedation.
Actions:	Competitively inhibits benzodiazepine-GABA receptor complex.
Side effects:	Seizures, dizziness, sweating, headache, blurred vision, anxiety, agitation, and increased muscle tone.
Comments:	Has been fatal in cases in which patients have shown signs of tricyclic overdose. Seizures are most common in these patients and those treated long term with benzodiazepines.
Dose:	In cases of suspected benzodiazepine overdose, give 0.2 mg IV over 30 seconds. Repeat after 30 seconds if desired level of consciousness is not obtained. Then repeat at 60-second intervals up to four times. In the event of re-sedation, repeated doses may be administered every 20 minutes. Maximum dose is 3 mg/hr.

Fluoxetine (Prozac)   *SSRI antidepressant*

Indications:	Depression, panic disorder, OCD.
Actions:	Blocks reuptake of serotonin into presynaptic neurons.
Side effects:	Agitation, insomnia, nausea, sexual dysfunction, akathisia, headache, and diarrhea.
Comments:	Half-life of fluoxetine and its metabolites is up to 9 days.
Interactions:	Increases levels of TCAs, carbamazepine, phenytoin, and some benzodiazepines. Do not use MAOI within 5 weeks of discontinuation of fluoxetine.
Dose:	Usual daily dose is 20 mg PO. May titrate up to a maximum of 80 mg daily. For OCD, higher doses may be necessary.

Fluphenazine (Prolixin)   *Antipsychotic*

Indications:	Psychosis, mania.
Actions:	Postsynaptic blockade of dopamine receptors.
Side effects:	Acute dystonia, parkinsonism, akathisia, NMS, tardive dyskinesia with long-term use, QT prolongation on ECG, postural hypotension, blurred vision, hyperprolactinemia, and exacerbation of glaucoma.
Comments:	High-potency antipsychotic with greater likelihood of extrapyramidal side effects and less sedative, anticholinergic, and hypotensive effects. May require 2 weeks of treatment for full antipsychotic effect. Depot form available. Use benztropine or diphenhydramine for acute dystonia.
Dose:	Initially, 0.5 to 10 mg PO daily. May increase to 20 mg daily. Use lower doses for elderly patients (1 to 2.5 mg

daily). For depot form, use 12.5 mg IM every 3 weeks for every 10 mg/day of oral fluphenazine equivalent.

Fluvoxamine (Luvox)   *SSRI antidepressant*

Indications:	Depression, OCD.
Actions:	Blocks presynaptic serotonin reuptake.
Side effects:	Nausea, somnolence, insomnia, sexual dysfunction.
Interactions:	Significant cytochrome interactions. Inhibits 1A2, 2C9, 2C19, 2D6, 3A3/4 isoenzymes. Increases levels of some benzodiazepines, calcium channel blockers, carbamazepine, clozapine, methadone, propranolol, theophylline, and TCAs.
Dose:	50 mg PO QD; titrate to maximum of 300 mg QD over several weeks.

Gabapentin (Neurontin)   *Anticonvulsant*

Indications:	Partial epilepsy, neuropathic pain, adjunctive treatment of bipolar disorder, anxiety.
Actions:	Unknown. Although structurally related to GABA, it has no effect on GABA receptors or on GABA uptake or degradation.
Side effects:	Somnolence, fatigue, ataxia, nausea, vomiting, dizziness.
Comments:	Few drug interactions, as drug is not hepatically metabolized. Amino acid transporter begins to saturate at doses >600 mg. Maalox will decrease absorption, so should give drug at least 2 hours after Maalox.
Dose:	Start at 300 mg PO TID, can titrate by 300 mg/day every day, usually up to 1800 to 2400 mg/day in divided doses. Effective doses have not been established, and doses over 3600 mg/day have been tolerated well.

Gabitril (See Tiagabine)

Guanfacine (Tenex)   *Antihypertensive*

Indications:	Attention-deficit disorder.
Actions:	Centrally acting alpha-2 agonism.
Side effects:	Dry mouth, sedation, weakness, dizziness, constipation.
Comments:	Rebound hypertension may occur 2 to 4 days after withdrawal but should resolve within 2 to 4 days.
Dose:	Start 0.5 mg/day and can increase by 0.5 mg every third day according to clinical response, up to 4 mg/day in divided doses.

Haldol (see Haloperidol)

Haloperidol (Haldol)   *Antipsychotic*

Indications:	Psychosis, mania, agitation.
Actions:	Postsynaptic blockade of dopamine receptors.
Side effects:	Acute dystonia, parkinsonism, akathisia, NMS, tardive dyskinesia with long-term use, QT interval prolonga-

tion on ECG, postural hypotension, blurred vision, hyperprolactinemia, exacerbation of glaucoma.

Comments: High-potency antipsychotic with greater likelihood of EPS and less sedative, anticholinergic, and hypotensive effects. May require 2 weeks of treatment for full antipsychotic effect. Depot form available. Use benztropine or diphenhydramine for acute dystonia. Useful in agitation due to dementia or delirium.

Dose: Initially, 0.5 to 10 mg PO daily. May increase to 20 mg daily. Use lower doses for elderly patients (1 to 2.5 mg daily). May give IV in ICU setting but should be pushed slowly to avoid torsades de pointes. For depot form use 150 mg IM every 4 weeks for every 10 mg/day of haloperidol equivalent.

Ibuprofen (Motrin)   *NSAID*

Indications: Inflammation due to arthritis and soft tissue injuries, analgesia.
Actions: Interferes with the actions of prostaglandins.
Side effects: Nausea and diarrhea. May compromise renal function in patients with renal impairment. Contraindicated in patients with the syndrome of aspirin sensitivity, nasal polyps, and bronchospasm. May result in increased lithium levels.
Dose: 200 to 400 mg PO TID to QID.

Imipramine (Tofranil)   *Tricyclic antidepressant*

Indications: Depression, panic disorder, enuresis, chronic pain syndromes.
Actions: Inhibits presynaptic reuptake of serotonin, norepinephrine, and dopamine.
Side effects: Sedation, postural hypotension, and anticholinergic effects. See Amitriptyline.
Comments: Less sedating with fewer anticholinergic effects than with amitriptyline, but more than with desipramine.
Dose: Start 25 mg PO HS and titrate slowly to usual daily dose of 150 to 200 mg. Doses range from 50 to 300 mg daily.

Inapsine (see **Droperidol**)

Inderal (see **Propranolol**)

Klonopin (see **Clonazepam**)

Lamictal (see **Lamotrigine**)

Lamotrigine (Lamictal)   *Anticonvulsant*

Indications: Bipolar disorder, especially mixed and depressed states. Refractory depression.

Actions:	Unknown.
Side effects:	Dizziness, nausea, headache, coordination difficulty, vomiting, and rash.
Comments:	Rash is common in about 10%. Because of risk of potentially life-threatening Stevens-Johnson syndrome (0.3 to 1.0%), drug should be discontinued at first sign of rash. Valproate will increase serum levels, so lower doses must be used in combination. Carbamazepine will decrease serum levels, so higher doses may be needed.
Dose:	As monotherapy, 25 mg PO QD for 1 week, then increase to 50 mg PO QD. Can increase by 50 mg/day every week until usual effective dose of 100 to 200 mg/day in divided doses is reached. If combined with valproate, 25 mg PO every other day for 2 weeks, then 25 mg PO QD for 2 weeks, then can increase 25 mg/day every week to effective dose. If combined with carbamazepine, start at 50 mg PO QD for 2 weeks, then 50 mg PO BID for 2 weeks, increasing 100 mg/day every 1 to 2 weeks to effective dose. Titration should be slow to avoid rash.

Levodopa-carbidopa (Sinemet) *Dopamine agonist*

Indications:	Parkinson's disease.
Actions:	Levodopa is converted to dopamine in the basal ganglia. Carbidopa inhibits the peripheral destruction of levodopa.
Side effects:	Anorexia, nausea, vomiting, abdominal pain, dysrhythmias, behavioral changes, orthostatic hypotension, psychosis, and involuntary movements.
Comments:	Side effects are common. Available in carbidopa-levodopa ratios of 1:4 and 1:10.
Dose:	Begin with 1 tablet 100 mg/10 mg or 100 mg/25 mg TID, increasing the dose until the desired response is obtained. Generally 75 mg/day of carbidopa is needed for full effect. Maximum dose is 8 tablets (800 mg/80 mg) daily divided TID or QID.

Librium (see **Chlordiazepoxide**)

Lithium carbonate (Eskalith) *Mood stabilizer*

Indications:	Bipolar disorder, antidepressant augmentation, cyclothymia, and schizoaffective disorder.
Actions:	Mechanism of action is unknown. May work on second-messenger systems.
Side effects:	Nausea, vomiting, diarrhea, anorexia, polyuria, polydipsia, rise in serum creatinine, edema, tremor, lethargy, fatigue, goiter, hypothyroidism, arrhythmias, T wave flattening or inversion on ECG, acne and psoriasis, weight gain, and hair loss.
Comments:	Before prescribing lithium, obtain history, physical, and baseline CBC, BUN/creatinine, T_4, T_3, TSH, and ECG.

Signs of lithium toxicity include new-onset GI symptoms, especially diarrhea, drowsiness, muscular weakness, lack of coordination, ataxia, and coarse tremor. Dehydration, low-sodium diets, diuretics can raise serum levels.

Dose: Begin 300 mg PO BID or TID. Obtain 12-hour trough serum levels every 5 days to adjust dose. Target serum levels for acute mania are 0.8 to 1.2 mEq/L; for maintenance, 0.6 to 1.0 mEq/L; and 0.5 to 0.8 mEq/L for antidepressant augmentation. Mild to moderate toxicity occurs between 1.5 and 2.0 mEq/L. Severe toxicity occurs at levels over 2.0 mEq/L.

Lorazepam (Ativan) *Benzodiazepine*

Indications: Anxiety, insomnia, agitation, alcohol withdrawal, muscle relaxation.

Actions: Depresses the CNS at the limbic and subcortical levels. Enhances the effect of the neurotransmitter GABA.

Side effects: Confusion, sedation, ataxia, respiratory depression at high doses. Use with care in patients with respiratory compromise, such as COPD. Paradoxical reaction of rage and disinhibition.

Comments: May cause dependence with prolonged use. Intermediate rate of onset and peak effect in 1 to 6 hours. Metabolism is less affected by aging and liver disease than with most other benzodiazepines. Metabolism is not cytochrome P450 dependent.

Dose: 0.5 to 1.0 mg PO QHS for sleep. For agitation, 1 to 2 mg PO/IM/IV PRN.

Loxapine (Loxitane) *Antipsychotic*

Indications: Psychosis, mania.

Actions: Postsynaptic blockade of dopamine receptors.

Side effects: Acute dystonia, parkinsonism, akathisia, NMS, tardive dyskinesia with long-term use, QT prolongation on ECG, postural hypotension, blurred vision, hyperprolactinemia, and exacerbation of glaucoma.

Comments: Use benztropine or diphenhydramine for acute dystonia. Medium-potency antipsychotic with greater sedative, hypotensive, and anticholinergic effects than with haloperidol and fluphenazine. Less likelihood of EPS than with higher-potency antipsychotics. Do not administer IV.

Dose: 10 mg PO or IM BID to QID, rapidly increasing to 60 to 100 mg PO QD for most patients. Maximum daily dose 250 mg.

Loxitane (see **Loxapine**)

Luminal (see **Phenobarbital**)

Luvox (see **Fluvoxamine**)

Maalox [Aluminum hydroxide–magnesium hydroxide]   *Antacid*

Indications: Pain due to peptic ulcer disease, reflux esophagitis, pro-
                 phylaxis of stress ulcer.
Actions: Buffers gastric acidity.
Side effects: Diarrhea and hypermagnesemia in renal failure.
Comments: Aluminum salts may cause constipation, and magnesium
                 salts cause diarrhea. The mixture attempts to balance
                 these effects. May bind and reduce absorption of tetra-
                 cycline, thyroxine, and other medications.
Dose: 30 to 60 mL PO every 2 to 4 hours PRN.

Mellaril [see **Thioridazine**]

Mesoridazine [Serentil]   *Antipsychotic*

Indications: Psychosis, mania.
Actions: Postsynaptic blockade of dopamine receptors.
Side effects: Acute dystonia, parkinsonism, akathisia, NMS, tardive
                 dyskinesia with long-term use, QT prolongation on
                 ECG, postural hypotension, blurred vision, hyperpro-
                 lactinemia, and exacerbation of glaucoma.
Comments: Low-potency antipsychotic with less likelihood of EPS
                 and greater sedative, anticholinergic, and hypoten-
                 sive effects.
Dose: 25 to 50 mg PO TID up to a maximum of 400 mg daily.
                 Usual effective dose 100 to 400 mg/day.

Methadone hydrochloride   *Narcotic*

Indications: Detoxification or maintenance treatment of narcotic ad-
                 diction.
Actions: Narcotic analgesic, splanchnic venodilation.
Side effects: Respiratory depression, dependence, light-headedness,
                 nausea, vomiting, constipation, and sweating.
Interactions: Levels increased by fluconazole, itraconazole, ketocona-
                 zole. Levels decreased by barbiturates, carbamazepine,
                 phenytoin, primidone, and rifampin.
Comments: Long half-life. In overdose, respiratory depression may
                 last 1 to 2 days, whereas administered antagonists may
                 reverse this effect for only several hours. Must monitor
                 patient who has overdosed for 1 to 2 days. Methadone
                 may be administered only by approved facilities.
Dose: Dose varies per patient requirement, usually 10 to 80
                 mg daily.

Methylphenidate [Ritalin]   *Psychostimulant*

Indications: Attention-deficit/hyperactivity disorder, narcolepsy.
Actions: Sympathomimetic amine, which causes release of norepi-
                 nephrine, dopamine, and serotonin from CNS nerve
                 terminals.
Side effects: Restlessness, tremor, insomnia, dysphoria, psychosis,
                 tachycardia, hypertension, rash, nausea, and vomiting.
Interactions: Avoid with MAOIs. In combination with venlafaxine,
                 NMS has been reported.

Comments: Prolonged use may lead to tolerance and dependence.
               May be used to augment antidepressants. Also used
               to treat apathy in the depressed, medically ill patient.
               Sustained release form has half-life of 8 hours but
               cannot be chewed or crushed.
Dose: 10 to 40 mg PO daily in divided doses. May increase to
               60 mg daily. Avoid half-strength and evening dosing.
               For children, start 0.3 mg/kg/dose at breakfast and
               lunch; titrate up to 2 mg/kg/day.

Mirtazapine (Remeron)   *Tetracyclic antidepressant*

Indications: Depression.
Actions: Speculated that selective alpha-2 antagonism increases
               noradrenergic and serotonin transmission.
Side effects: Sedation, weight gain, dizziness. Agranulocytosis re-
               ported in two patients, neutropenia in one.
Interactions: Contraindicated within 2 weeks of MAOI.
Comments: More highly sedating at low doses.
Dose: Start 15 mg PO QHS (7.5 mg in elderly); increase up to
               45 mg QHS. Typical dose 30 mg QHS.

Moban (see Molindone)

Molindone (Moban)   *Antipsychotic*

Indications: Psychosis, mania.
Actions: Postsynaptic blockade of dopamine receptors.
Side effects: Acute dystonia, parkinsonism, akathisia, NMS, tardive
               dyskinesia with long-term use, QT interval prolonga-
               tion on ECG, postural hypotension, blurred vision,
               hyperprolactinemia, and exacerbation of glaucoma.
Comments: Medium-potency antipsychotic with less likelihood of
               EPS and greater sedative, anticholinergic, and hypo-
               tensive effects than with haloperidol and fluphenazine.
               May require 2 weeks of treatment for full antipsychotic
               effect. The only antipsychotic that is not associated
               with weight gain.
Dose: Start 50 to 75 mg PO in three or four divided doses,
               increase to 100 mg/day in 3 to 4 days, and titrate up
               to a maximum of 225 mg daily.

Morphine sulfate   *Narcotic analgesic*

Indications: Moderate to severe pain, pulmonary edema.
Actions: Binds opiate receptors in CNS.
Side effects: Respiratory depression, hypotension, nausea, and vom-
               iting.
Comments: 10 mg morphine IM/SC = 100 mg meperidine IM/
               SC. Phenothiazines may decrease efficacy of morphine.
               Narcotic effect may be enhanced by TCAs and other
               CNS depressants.

Dose: For chest pain due to coronary ischemia, 2 to 4 mg IV
                        every 5 to 10 minutes to a maximum of 10 to 12 mg.
                        For pain, 2 to 15 mg IV/IM/SC every 4 hours PRN.

Naloxone (Narcan)   *Narcotic antagonist*

Indications: Respiratory depression due to narcotics.
Actions: Probably competes with opioid receptor sites.
Side effects: Dysphoria, agitation, seizures, tachycardia, nausea, vom-
                        iting, and increased blood pressure.
Comments: The patient should be continuously monitored for re-
                        emergence of respiratory depression as naloxone's
                        half-life is short compared with that of most opioids.
Dose: 0.4 to 2 mg IV as initial dose. May be repeated at 2- to
                        3-minute intervals up to a maximum dose of 10 mg.
                        If no response, one should question the diagnosis of
                        narcotic toxicity.

Naltrexone (ReVia, Trexan)   *Opioid antagonist*

Indications: Alcohol dependence, opioid dependence, prevention of
                        self-mutilation.
Actions: Opioid antagonist.
Side effects: Hepatic toxicity, insomnia, anxiety, nausea, and head-
                        ache.
Comments: Should not be started until verified that the patient has
                        been opioid free for 7 to 10 days and is without evi-
                        dence of liver damage (e.g., normal LFTs).
Dose: 50 mg PO daily.

Narcan (see **Naloxone**)

Nardil (see **Phenelzine**)

Navane (see **Thiothixene**)

Nefazodone (Serzone)   *Antidepressant*

Indications: Depression.
Actions: 5-HT$_2$ antagonist; also inhibits serotonin and norepi-
                        nephrine reuptake.
Side effects: Sedation, nausea, dizziness, dry mouth, blurred vision,
                        constipation.
Interactions: Significant inhibition of the cytochrome P450 3A4 sub-
                        type. Contraindicated with astemizole, terfenadine,
                        and pimozide. Avoid with MAOIs and triazolam. Ne-
                        fazodone increases fluoxetine levels. Administration
                        with SSRIs may cause serotonin syndrome. Has been
                        associated with rhabdomyolysis when given with
                        HMG-CoA reductase inhibitors, especially lovastatin
                        and simvastatin.
Comments: Less alpha-adrenergic blockade than with its more sedat-
                        ing relative, trazodone.

Dose: Start 50 to 100 mg PO BID and titrate over several days
                   to 150 to 300 mg BID.

Neurontin (see **Gabapentin**)

Nortriptyline (Pamelor)   *Tricyclic antidepressant*

Indications: Depression, chronic pain.
Actions: Inhibits norepinephrine and serotonin reuptake.
Side effects: Orthostatic hypotension, anticholinergic effects. See Am-
                   itriptyline.
Interactions: Contraindicated within 2 weeks of MAOI. Levels may
                   be increased by some SSRIs.
Comments: Therapeutic blood level 50 to 150 ng/mL; less likely than
                   other TCAs to cause orthostasis. Monitor ECGs.
Dose: Start 25 mg PO QHS and titrate to 75 to 100 mg QD.
                   Maximum of 150 mg QD.

Olanzapine (Zyprexa)   *Antipsychotic*

Indications: Psychosis, acute mania.
Actions: D_1, D_2, D_4, and 5-HT_2 antagonism.
Side effects: Drowsiness, dry mouth, akathisia, dizziness, and consti-
                   pation. Weight gain and orthostatic hypotension can
                   occur.
Comments: Long-term weight gain can be significant. EPS less com-
                   mon than with typical antipsychotics at usual doses.
                   Case reports of diabetes associated with administra-
                   tion.
Dose: 5 to 10 mg PQ QHS; increase by 5 mg every week to
                   maximum dose of 20 mg.

Orap (see **Pimozide**)

Oxazepam (Serax)   *Benzodiazepine*

Indications: Insomnia, anxiety.
Actions: Depresses the CNS at the limbic and subcortical levels.
                   Enhances the effect of the neurotransmitter GABA.
Side effects: Confusion, drowsiness, and hangover effect. Respiratory
                   depression. Use with care in patients with respiratory
                   compromise, such as COPD.
Comments: Risk of dependence. Useful in elderly patients or those
                   with cirrhosis who might have compromised liver
                   function; peak levels in 1 to 4 hours.
Dose: 15 mg PO QHS for insomnia. For anxiety, 10 to 30 mg
                   TID.

Pamelor (see **Nortriptyline**)

Parlodel (see **Bromocriptine**)

Parnate (see **Tranylcypromine**)

Paroxetine (Paxil)   *SSRI antidepressant*

Indications: Depression, panic disorder, OCD.
Actions: Inhibits serotonin reuptake.
Side effects: Nausea, sedation, insomnia, and sexual dysfunction.
Interactions: Can increase levels of antiarrhythmics, cimetidine and
                 TCAs. May increase INR with warfarin. May cause
                 serotonin syndrome with other serotonergic agents.
                 Contraindicated within 2 weeks of MAOI.
Comments: More sedating than other SSRIs. Use higher doses in
                 OCD. Can be associated with flu-like withdrawal
                 symptoms if abruptly discontinued.
Dose: 20 mg PO QD up to a maximum of 80 mg daily.

Paxil (see **Paroxetine**)

Pemoline (Cylert)   *Stimulant*

Indications: Attention-deficit/hyperactivity disorder, as an adjunct to
                 refractory depression.
Actions: Causes dopamine release in the CNS.
Side effects: Insomnia, irritability, and nervousness.
Comments: Drug is associated with fatal hepatotoxicity. LFT blood
                 samples should be drawn at baseline and periodically
                 thereafter. Contraindicated in patients with impaired
                 hepatic function.
Dose: Start at 37.5 mg PO QD and increase by 18.75 mg/day
                 every week. Usual effective dose is 56.25 to 75 mg;
                 maximum dose of 112.5 mg daily.

Perphenazine (Trilafon)   *Antipsychotic*

Indications: Psychosis, agitation.
Actions: Postsynaptic blockade of CNS dopamine receptors.
Side effects: Dystonia, drowsiness, dizziness, dry mouth, and consti-
                 pation. Akathisia, pseudoparkinsonism, NMS, tardive
                 dyskinesia also possible.
Comments: Greater likelihood of EPS and less sedation and anticho-
                 linergic side effects.
Dose: 8 to 16 mg PO BID, TID, or QID up to a maximum of 64
                 mg daily. 5 to 10 mg IM can be used for agitation.

Phenelzine (Nardil)   *MAOI antidepressant*

Indications: Atypical depression, severe depression, PTSD.
Actions: Inhibits MAO, increasing norepinephrine and serotonin.
Side effects: Orthostatic hypotension, edema, weight gain, and in-
                 somnia.
Interactions: May cause hypoglycemia with oral hypoglycemics. With
                 other antidepressants and carbamazepine, causes sero-
                 tonin syndrome. Autonomic instability with opiates.
                 Contraindicated with sympathomimetics, CNS depres-
                 sants, meperidine, bupropion, buspirone, general or
                 spinal anesthesia, dextromethorphan. May exaggerate
                 effect of antihypertensives. Should wait 2 weeks after
                 discontinuation of SSRIs, 5 weeks after discontinuation
                 of fluoxetine before starting phenelzine.

Comments: Risk of hypertensive crisis if tyramine-containing foods
                are ingested, such as red wine, cheese, smoked or
                pickled fish, beef or chicken liver, dried sausage, fava
                or broad bean pods, yeast vitamin supplements. Avoid
                foods high in tryptophan, dopamine, chocolate, or caf-
                feine.
Dose: Patients should be given a trial dose of 15 mg on the
                initial day of treatment, with titration to 15 mg PO
                TID during the first week by 15 mg/day.

Phenobarbital (Luminal)   *Barbiturate*

Indications: Seizure disorder, sedation, insomnia.
Actions: Sedative, hypnotic.
Side effects: Drowsiness, hypotension, and respiratory depression.
Comments: Not generally used for insomnia currently owing to high
                abuse potential. In overdose, look for slurred speech,
                ataxia, and nystagmus.
Dose: 60 mg PO BID or TID.

Phenytoin (Dilantin)   *Anticonvulsant*

Indications: Seizures.
Actions: Promotes neuronal sodium efflux, stabilizing neuron
                membrane.
Side effects: Dizziness, nystagmus, slurred speech, tremor, rash, Ste-
                vens-Johnson syndrome, blood dyscrasias, gingival
                hyperplasia, periarteritis nodosa.
Interactions: Psychiatric medications that increase phenytoin levels
                include chlordiazepoxide, diazepam, disulfiram, estro-
                gens, trazodone. Medications that decrease phenytoin
                levels include carbamazepine, reserpine, molindone.
                Medications that may increase or decrease phenytoin
                levels include phenobarbital and valproate. Acute al-
                cohol intake raises levels; chronic intake decreases lev-
                els. TCAs may potentiate seizures with phenytoin.
Comment: Effective serum level usually 10 to 20 μg/mL and must
                be monitored.
Dose: Start 100 mg PO TID; increase if needed to therapeutic
                blood level.

Pimozide (Orap)   *Antipsychotic*

Indications: Tourette's syndrome, psychosis.
Actions: Postsynaptic blockade of CNS dopamine receptors.
Side effects: Extrapyramidal symptoms, prolongation of QT interval,
                T wave changes.
Comments: High-potency antipsychotic. Contraindicated in patients
                with a history of arrhythmia or other drugs that pro-
                long QT interval. Contraindicated with macrolide anti-
                biotics, such as clarithromycin, erythromycin, azithro-
                mycin, dirithromycin, azole antifungal agents, and
                protease inhibitors.
Dosage: 0.5 to 1 mg PO BID; may increase every other day to
                maximum dose of 0.2 mg/kg or 10 mg.

Prochloperazine (Compazine)   *Antiemetic, antipsychotic*

Indications: Severe nausea, vomiting, psychosis.
Actions: Blocks D_2, muscarinic, and histaminic receptors.
Side effects: Pseudoparkinsonism, akathisia, dystonic reaction, confusion, NMS, tardive dyskinesia, anticholinergic effects, orthostatic hypotension, blood dyscrasias.
Interactions: Increases phenytoin levels, decreases warfarin levels. Additive side effects with other typical antipsychotics.
Comments: Rarely used for psychiatric purposes.
Dose: 5 to 10 mg PO TID or 25 mg per rectum BID.

Prolixin (see **Fluphenazine**)

Propranolol (Inderal)   *Beta-blocker*

Indications: Akathisia, situational anxiety, intermittent explosive disorder.
Actions: Beta-adrenergic blocker.
Side effects: Bradycardia and hypotension.
Comments: High doses usually needed to control violent outbursts.
Dose: 10 to 80 mg PO QD (may give in divided doses); start 10 mg TID for akathisia and increase as tolerated until effective dose is reached.

Quetiapine (Seroquel)   *Antipsychotic*

Indications: Psychosis.
Actions: $5\text{-}HT_2$, D_1, D_2 antagonism.
Side effects: Somnolence, dizziness, headache, orthostatic hypotension. NMS possible.
Comments: Risk of orthostasis greatest during initial 3 to 5 days and when dose is increased. Lower risk for hyperprolactinemia or EPS than with other antipsychotics. Slit-lamp examinations are officially recommended by the manufacturer at baseline and every 6 months. Cataracts developed only in premarketing studies with dogs, however, and no causal relationship to cataracts in humans has been shown.
Dosage: Start at 25 mg PO BID; increase by 25 to 50 mg BID every 2 to 3 days to usual effective dose of 300 to 400 mg day. Maximum dose is 750 mg PO QD.

Remeron (see **Mirtazapine**)

Restoril (see **Temazepam**)

Revia (see **Naltrexone**)

Risperdal (see **Risperidone**)

Risperidone (Risperdal)   *Antipsychotic*

Indications: Psychosis.
Actions: $5\text{-}HT_2$ and D_2 antagonist.

Side effects:	Orthostatic hypotension, sedation, dizziness, weight gain, dystonia, NMS, akathisia, and pseudoparkinsonism.
Comments:	With increasing dose, risk of EPS increases; usual effective daily dose is 4 to 8 mg daily. Increased likelihood of akathisia when given with valproic acid.
Dose:	Start 0.5 to 1 mg PO BID and increase by 1 mg per week to a maximum of 16 mg daily. Effective dose usually 2 to 6 mg/day.

Ritalin [see **Methylphenidate**]

Romazicon [see **Flumazenil**]

Selegiline [Eldepryl]   *Antiparkinsonian agent*

Indications:	Adjunctive treatment in Parkinson's disease.
Actions:	Inhibits MAO B (selective inhibitor).
Side effects:	Severe agitation, confusion, depression, and hallucinations.
Comments:	At doses above 10 mg daily, risks of nonselective MAO inhibition increase. Otherwise only rare reactions with tyramine or SSRIs are reported. Should avoid use of SSRIs or TCAs for 14 days after discontinuation of selegiline.
Dose:	5 mg PO BID.

Serax [see **Oxazepam**]

Serentil [see **Mesoridazine**]

Seroquel [see **Quetiapine**]

Sertraline [Zoloft]   *SSRI antidepressant*

Indications:	Depression, panic disorder.
Actions:	Inhibits presynaptic serotonin reuptake.
Side effects:	Nausea, diarrhea, agitation, and sexual dysfunction.
Interactions:	Mild elevation of TCA and antiarrhythmic levels. Contraindicated within 2 weeks of MAOI.
Comments:	Less sedating than paroxetine, less activating than fluoxetine.
Dose:	50 mg PO QD up to a maximum daily dose of 200 mg.

Serzone [see **Nefazodone**]

Sinemet [see **Levodopa-carbidopa**]

Sonata [see **Zaleplon**]

Symmetrel [see **Amantadine**]

Synthroid [see **Thyroxine**]

Tacrine (Cognex)   *Acetylcholinesterase inhibitor*

Indications:	Treatment of cognitive impairment associated with early Alzheimer's disease.
Actions:	Reversible nonselective acetylcholinesterase inhibitor.
Side effects:	Reversible elevation of liver enzymes is fairly common. Nausea, vomiting, diarrhea, dyspepsia, myalgia, anorexia, and ataxia.
Comments:	Risk of hepatotoxicity limits its use.
Dose:	Start at 10 mg PO QID; and can increase by 40 mg/day in divided doses every 4 weeks to maximum of 160 mg/day as tolerated.

Tegretol (see **Carbamazepine**)

Temazepam (Restoril)   *Benzodiazepine*

Indications:	Insomnia.
Actions:	Sedative, hypnotic.
Side effects:	Confusion, drowsiness, dependence, and hangover effect.
Comments:	Peak levels at 3 hours.
Dose:	15 to 30 mg PO QHS; 7.5 mg in elderly.

Tenex (see **Guanfacine**)

Thioridazine (Mellaril)   *Antipsychotic*

Indications:	Psychosis, behavioral problems in children, agitation.
Actions:	Postsynaptic blockade of CNS dopamine receptors.
Side effects:	Orthostatic hypotension, dry mouth, constipation, dizziness, drowsiness, retrograde ejaculation, NMS, tardive dyskinesia.
Comments:	At doses exceeding 800 mg daily, risk for retinal pigmentary changes increases; low-potency antipsychotic with less risk of dystonia and EPS.
Dose:	50 to 100 mg PO TID up to a maximum daily dose of 800 mg. Effective daily dose usually between 100 and 600 mg/day.

Thiothixene (Navane)   *Antipsychotic*

Indications:	Psychosis.
Actions:	Postsynaptic blockade of CNS dopamine receptors.
Side effects:	Acute dystonia, parkinsonism, akathisia, NMS, tardive dyskinesia with long-term use, QT interval prolongation on ECG, postural hypotension, blurred vision, hyperprolactinemia, exacerbation of glaucoma.
Comments:	IM form available; high-potency antipsychotic.
Dose:	Start 2 mg PO TID and increase to a maximum daily dose of 60 mg. Usual effective dose is 20 to 30 mg/day.

Thorazine (see **Chlorpromazine**)

Thyroxine (Synthroid) *Thyroid hormone*

Indications:	Hypothyroidism and augmentation of antidepressants.
Actions:	Mechanism of action for augmentation is not known.
Side effects:	In overdose, similar to thyrotoxicosis. May cause transient hair loss.
Comments:	Before lithium therapy, obtain baseline TSH, T_3, and T_4 levels.
Dose:	25 to 50 μg PO QD for augmentation in depression. Change in dose not reflected in TSH for approximately 1 month. May use up to 300 μg PO QD for hypothyroidism.

Tiagabine (Gabitril) *Anticonvulsant*

Indications:	Partial epilepsy; presumptively used in bipolar and schizoaffective disorders.
Actions:	Uncertain; enhances activity of GABA in vitro.
Side effects:	Dizziness, somnolence, nausea, weakness. Potential for rash, including Stevens-Johnson syndrome.
Comments:	Very limited evidence for use in psychiatric disorders.
Dose:	Start at 4 mg PO QD, and increase by 4 mg per day in second week. May then increase by 4 to 8 mg/day each week until a maximum daily dose of 32 mg/day in two to four divided doses.

Topamax (see **Topiramate**)

Topiramate (Topamax) *Anticonvulsant*

Indications:	Bipolar disorder.
Actions:	Unknown.
Side effects:	Somnolence, dizziness, vision problems, unsteadiness, speech problems, psychomotor slowing, paresthesia, nervousness, nausea, memory problems, tremor, confusion.
Comments:	Psychomotor slowing and cognitive side effects such as memory problems and confusion are most likely to cause discontinuation, but side effects generally diminish a few days after a dose increase. Weight loss can be seen, and drug can be used to help reverse weight gain caused by other mood stabilizers. Kidney stones were seen in 1.5% of patients in premarketing studies, as drug has weak carbonic anhydrase activity. Increased water intake should be recommended to prevent kidney stones.
Dose:	Start at 12.5 to 25 mg PO QD, and titrate by 12.5 to 25 mg/day every week to an effective dose of 100 to 200 mg/day, although some patients require 400 mg in divided doses, especially if used as monotherapy.

Tranxene (see **Clorazepate**)

Tranylcypromine (Parnate)   *MAOI antidepressant*

Indications:	Atypical depression, severe depression.
Actions:	Inhibits MAO, increasing norepinephrine and serotonin.
Side effects:	Orthostatic hypotension, edema, weight gain, and insomnia.
Interactions:	May cause hypoglycemia with oral hypoglycemics. With other antidepressants and carbamazepine, causes serotonin syndrome. Autonomic instability with opiates. Contraindicated with sympathomimetics, CNS depressants, meperidine, bupropion, buspirone, general or spinal anesthesia, dextromethorphan. May exaggerate effect of antihypertensives. Should wait 2 weeks after discontinuation of SSRIs, 5 weeks after discontinuation of fluoxetine before starting MAOI.
Comments:	Risk of hypertensive crisis if tyramine-containing foods are ingested, such as red wine, cheese, smoked or pickled fish, beef or chicken liver, dried sausage, fava or broad bean pods, yeast vitamin supplements. Avoid foods high in tryptophan, dopamine, chocolate, or caffeine.
Dose:	Begin with a trial dose of 10 mg daily, and increase to 30 mg per day in divided doses during the first week.

Trazodone (Desyrel)   *Antidepressant*

Indications:	Depression, insomnia.
Actions:	Postsynaptic serotonin agonist; also inhibits serotonin reuptake.
Side effects:	Sedation and orthostatic hypotension; rarely, priapism in males.
Interactions:	Avoid use with MAOIs. May elevate digoxin and phenytoin levels and alter PT/INR in patients taking warfarin.
Comments:	Owing to high level of sedation, is most useful as a sleep agent.
Dose:	For sleep, 50 to 100 mg PO QHS; for depression, 200 to 300 mg daily in divided doses up to a maximum daily dose of 600 mg.

Trexan (see **Naltrexone**)

Trilafon (see **Perphenazine**)

Valium (see **Diazepam**)

Valproic acid (Depakene, Depakote)   *Anticonvulsant*

Indications:	Acute mania, bipolar disorder.
Actions:	Unknown.
Side effects:	Nausea, vomiting, sedation, dizziness, weakness, tremor, weight gain, alopecia.
Comments:	Divalproex sodium (Depakote) less likely to cause GI upset; optimal blood level is 50 to 125 µg/mL. Contraindicated in patients with history of hepatic disease.

Potentially fatal hepatoxicity is more likely in infants and can be preceded by malaise, weakness, lethargy, facial edema, anorexia, and vomiting. Frequent LFT monitoring is recommended in first 6 months. Risk of thrombocytopenia warrants baseline CBC every 1 to 2 weeks for first 2 months and every 6 months after. Discontinue if platelets <100,000/mm^3.

Dose: 250 mg PO BID or TID for 3 to 4 days, then increasing to 500 mg PO BID and checking levels every 3 to 4 days. Therapeutic doses range from 750 to 2500 mg/day. Rapid loading in acute mania can be done using 20 mg/kg. This can attain therapeutic dose more quickly but with more side effects.

Venlafaxine (Effexor; *Antidepressant*
extended release:
Effexor XR)

Indications:	Depression, generalized anxiety disorder.
Actions:	Inhibits serotonin and norepinephrine reuptake.
Side effects:	Anxiety, nausea, sedation, and dizziness. At higher doses, may elevate BP.
Interactions:	Contraindicated within 2 weeks of MAOI.
Comments:	Sustained release form (XR) better tolerated and more commonly used. Decreased clearance in hepatic and renal dysfunction warrants lower dose.
Dose:	Sustained release: 37.5 mg PO QD to start, titrate up to 225 mg QD, usual dose 150 QD. Immediate release: 75 to 225 mg a day in divided doses; maximum daily dose 375 mg.

Warfarin (Coumadin) *Anticoagulant*

Indications:	Prophylaxis and/or treatment of venous thrombosis.
Actions:	Inhibits synthesis of vitamin K–dependent clotting factors.
Side effects:	Hemorrhage, skin and organ necrosis, hepatitis.
Interactions:	Psychiatric drugs that increase PT/INR include chloral hydrate, disulfiram, fluoxetine, fluvoxamine, thyroxine, methylphenidate, paroxetine, prednisone, sertraline, and valproate, as well as vitamin E. Drugs that decrease PT/INR include barbiturates, chlordiazepoxide, carbamazepine, trazodone.
Comments:	Usual therapeutic INR 2.0 to 3.0.
Dose:	Individualized by INR; typically 2 to 10 mg PO QD.

Xanax (see Alprazolam)

Zaleplon (Sonata) *Nonbenzodiazepine hypnotic*

Indications:	Insomnia.
Actions:	Not a benzodiazepine, but binds subunit of GABA-A receptor complex.
Side effects:	Sedation, dizziness.
Interactions:	Cimetidine increases zaleplon levels.
Comments:	Rapid onset action. Recent high-fat meal, 3A4 inducers may reduce effectiveness.
Dose:	5 to 10 mg PO QHS.

Zoloft (see **Sertraline**)

Zolpidem (Ambien)   *Nonbenzodiazepine hypnotic*

Indications:	Insomnia.
Actions:	Sedative, hypnotic.
Side effects:	Nausea, vomiting, diarrhea, headache, and dizziness.
Comments:	Peak levels in 1 to 2 hours; shares some of the pharmacologic properties of the benzodiazepines.
Dose:	10 mg PO QHS; 5 mg PO QHS for elderly patients.

Zyban (see **Bupropion**)

Zyprexa (see **Olanzapine**)

INDEX

Note: Page numbers in *italics* refer to illustrations; page numbers followed by t refer to tables.

A

Abandonment. See also *Neglect.*
  of elders, 254
Abuse, emotional, 251, 253
  indicators of, 45, 249–251
  mandatory reporting of, 45, 123, 254
  of children. See *Child abuse.*
  of elders. See *Elder abuse.*
  of women. See *Women, abuse of.*
  physical. See *Physical abuse.*
  sexual, 251, 253. See also *Rape victim.*
  substance, 125–134. See also *Intoxication.*
  suspected, referrals for, 254
  telephone hotlines for, 16, 255
  victims of, seclusion and restraint of, 20
Acetaminophen (Tylenol), 257
L-Acetyl-α-methadol (LAMM), for opiate withdrawal, 144, 145
Acquired immunodeficiency syndrome (AIDS), in substance abusers, 136, 145
  manifesting as psychiatric disorder, 52, 83, 215
  suicidal ideation with, 79
  telephone hotlines for, 16, 255
Acute intermittent porphyria, manifesting as psychiatric disorder, 83, 215
Addictive behaviors, telephone hotlines for, 255–256
Addison's disease (adrenal cortical insufficiency), manifesting as psychiatric disorder, 215
Administrative consultation, for treatment consent, 30, 31–32
Admission, of patient, consultations for, 30–32
  following child and adolescent evaluation, 45

Admission *(Continued)*
  types of, 31
Admission orders, 232
Adolescent(s), as runaways, telephone hotlines for, 255
Adolescent evaluation, 40–46
  chart review for, 42–43
  for aggression/homicidal ideation, 44
  for agitation, medication dosages for, 45–46
    seclusion and restraint of, 20, 45
  for psychosis, 44
  for suicide, 43–44
  hospitalization following, 45
  initial approach to, 41–42
  management following, 44–46
  selective history in, 42–43
  telephone consultation for, 40–41
  threat to life in, 42
Adrenal cortical insufficiency (Addison's disease), manifesting as psychiatric disorder, 215
Adrenergic receptor blockers, adverse effects of, 246
Adult protection services, 254
Affect, in mental status examination, 212
Agitation, 49–56. See also *Violence.*
  causes of, 50–52
  definition of, 49
  in children and adolescents, 45–46
  in difficult patient, 34, 36
  in rape victims, 119
  laboratory tests for, 54–55
  management of, continued, 54–55
    drugs for, 55–56
    initial, 53–54
  quick look test for, 53

Oxcarbazepine, for seizures, 193

P

Pain, chest, 167–173. See also *Chest pain.*
  chronic, insomnia with, 152, 153t
Pain management, with nausea and vomiting, 174, 177
Pancreatic carcinoma, manifesting as psychiatric disorder, 219
Papilledema, disc changes seen in, 163, *164*
  nuchal rigidity with, 163
Parathyroid disorder(s), manifesting as psychiatric disorder, 217, 218
Parents Anonymous, 255
Parkinsonism, drug-induced, 105
  clinical features of, 100, 105
  management of, 105–106
Parkinson's disease, insomnia in, 153t
Paroxetine (Paxil), 276
  adverse effects of, 235
Paroxysmal events, nonepileptic, seizures *vs.*, 186
Partial (focal) seizures, 186–187
  drug therapy for, 192t
Patient, admission of, 30–31
  involuntary, 31–32
  agitated, 49–56. See also *Agitation.*
  anxious, 57–65. See also *Anxiety.*
  competency of, assessment of, 27–30
  confidentiality of, exceptions to, 32–33
  difficult, 34–39. See also *Difficult patient.*
  discharge of, 32
  establishing rapport with, 10–11
  intoxicated, 125–134. See also *Intoxication.*
  involuntary treatment of, 31–32
  mute, 107–117. See also *Mutism.*
  psychotic, 81–86. See also *Psychosis.*
  seclusion and restraint of, 18–26. See also *Seclusion and restraint.*
  self-identification of, in telephone consultations, 14–15, 17

Patient *(Continued)*
  suicidal, 73–80. See also *Suicidal patient.*
  support system of. See *Support system.*
  violent, 66–72. See also *Violence.*
Patient chart, documentation of, seclusion and restraint in, 24–25
  review of, 9, 10
Patient interview, during consultation, 11
Pemoline (Cylert), 276
  adverse effects of, 247
Pentobarbital (Nembutal), coma, for seizures, 191
  for CNS depressant withdrawal, 142–143
Peptic ulcer disease, chest pain with, 168, 171, 172
  management of, 173
Perceptual disorder(s), in mental status examination, 212, 213
Perphenazine (Trilafon), 276
  adverse effects of, 241
Phencyclidine hydrochloride (PCP) intoxication, 126, 131–132
  psychosis from, 111
Phenelzine (Nardil), 276–277
  adverse effects of, 238
Phenobarbital (Luminal), 277
  for CNS depressant withdrawal, 143
  for seizures, 191, 192t, 193t
Phenoxybenzamine, for hypertensive crisis, 163
Phentolamine, for hypertensive crisis, 163
Phenytoin (Dilantin), 277
  for seizures, 140, 192t, 193t
Pheochromocytoma, manifesting as psychiatric disorder, 219
Physical abuse, in special populations, 122–124
  indicators of, 249–251
  of child, 45, 122–123, 250
  of elders, 252–253
  of women, 118–123, 255
  telephone hotlines for, 16, 255
Physical neglect, indicators of, 250
Physician, communicating with, 12–13
  consultant relationship with, 6–7